Contributors

Editors

Hugh Freeman
University of Manchester School of Medicine, Hope Hospital, Eccles Old Road, Salford M6 8HD, UK

Yvonne Rue
45 New High Street, Oxford OX3 7AL, UK

Contributors

Anthony Clare *(Chairman)*
Department of Psychological Medicine, St Bartholomew's Hospital Medical College, London EC1A 7BE, UK

Roger Higgs
Department of General Practice Studies, King's College School of Medicine and Dentistry, Denmark Hill, London SE5 9RS, UK

Malcolm Lader
Department of Psychiatry, Institute of Psychiatry, De Crespigny Park, London SE5 8AP, UK

Karl Rickels
Department of Psychiatry, University of Pennsylvania, Philadelphia, Pennsylvania 19104, USA

Edward Schweizer
Department of Psychiatry, University of Pennsylvania, Philadelphia, Pennsylvania 19104, USA

David Taylor
Association of the British Pharmaceutical Industry, 12 Whitehall, London SW1A 2DY, UK

Paul Turner
Department of Clinical Pharmacology, St Bartholomew's Hospital, London EC1A 7BE, UK

Peter Tyrer
Mapperley Hospital, Nottingham NG3 6AA, UK

Frank Wells
Association of the British Pharmaceutical Industry, 12 Whitehall, London SW1A 2DY, UK

Paul Williams
General Practice Research Unit, Institute of Psychiatry, De Crespigny Park, London SE5 8AF, UK

Discussants

Michael Beary
  Department of Psychiatry, St George's Hospital Medical School, London SW17 0RE, UK

Tom Christie
  Director of Medical Corporate Affairs, Wyeth International

Sandra File
  MRC Neuropharmacology Research Group, School of Pharmacy, University of London, London WC1N 1AX, UK

Norman Imlah
  Department of Psychiatry, All Saints Hospital, Lodge Road, Birmingham B18 5SD, UK

John Marks
  Mersey Regional Drug Dependency Service, Liverpool L1 9BX, UK

John L. Reed
  Principal Medical Officer, Department of Health and Social Security, Alexander Fleming House, London SE1 6BY, UK

David Wheatley
  Psychopharmacology Research Group, The Stress Clinic, Maudsley Hospital, Denmark Hill, London SE5 8AZ

International Congress and Symposium Series

Editor-in-Chief: Hugh L'Etang

The benzodiazepines in current clinical practice
Proceedings of a symposium sponsored by Wyeth Laboratories, held in London 20 January 1987

International Congress and Symposium Series
Number 114

The benzodiazepines in current clinical practice

Edited by
Hugh Freeman
Yvonne Rue

Royal Society of Medicine Services
London   New York
1987

Royal Society of Medicine Services Limited
1 Wimpole Street   London W1M 8AE
7 East 60th Street   New York   NY 10022

©1987 Royal Society of Medicine Services Limited

All rights reserved. No part of this book may be reproduced in any form by photostat, microfilm, or any other means, without written permission from the publishers.

This publication is copyright under the Berne Convention and the International Copyright Convention. All rights reserved. Apart from any fair dealing under the UK Copyright Act 1956, Part 1, Section 7, no part of this publication may be reproduced, stored in a retrieval system or transmitted in any form or by any means without the prior permission of the Honorary Editors, Royal Society of Medicine.

These proceedings are published by Royal Society of Medicine Services Ltd with financial support from the sponsor. The contributors are responsible for the scientific content and for the views expressed, which are not necessarily those of the sponsor, of the editor of the series or of the volume, of the Royal Society of Medicine or of Royal Society of Medicine Services Ltd. Distribution has been in accordance with the wishes of the sponsor but a copy is available to any Fellow of the Society at a privileged price.

British Library Cataloguing in Publication Data
The benzodiazepines in current clinical practice.—
 (The Royal Society of Medicine international congress
 and symposium series; 114).
 1. Benzodiazepines
 I. Freeman, Hugh   II. Rue, Yvonne
 III. Series
 615'.7882   RM666.B42
 ISBN 0-905958-45-4

Editorial and production services by Yvonne Rue, 45 New High Street, Oxford OX3 7AL
Phototypeset by Dobbie Typesetting Limited, Plymouth, Devon
Printed in Great Britain at the Alden Press, Oxford

Contents

List of Contributors	v
Introductory remarks ANTHONY CLARE	1
Benefits and risks of benzodiazepines PETER TYRER	3
Discussion	11
Current usage of benzodiazepines in Britain DAVID TAYLOR	13
Discussion	17
Long-term benzodiazepine use in general practice PAUL WILLIAMS	19
Discussion	32
Psychiatric indications for benzodiazepines KARL RICKELS and EDWARD SCHWEIZER	35
Discussion	41
Adjustment disorders and environmental change — benzodiazepines and other treatments in general practice ROGER HIGGS	43
Benzodiazepines and the general physician PAUL TURNER	47
Discussion	51
Long-term benzodiazepine use and psychological functioning MALCOLM LADER	55
Discussion	69
General discussion	71
Chairman's summing up ANTHONY CLARE	81

Introductory remarks

ANTHONY CLARE

*Department of Psychological Medicine,
St Bartholomew's Hospital Medical College, London EC1A 7BE, UK*

The organizers of this Symposium entitled 'The benzodiazepines in current clinical practice' wanted to bring together representatives of those areas of medicine in which the benzodiazepines are currently most commonly used—general practice, general medicine, and psychiatry—as well as contributions from epidemiology, pharmacology, clinical medicine and biochemistry.

The development of the benzodiazepines and their clinical proliferation must be one of the landmarks of post-war clinical medicine; the remarkable growth in their popularity, which led to a peak of some 30 million prescriptions a year in the UK by the end of the 1970s, has been attributed variously to the relative safety, efficacy, and cheapness of benzodiazepines. Certainly, when compared to their anxiolytic predecessors—bromides, alcohol and the barbiturates—they do appear to have many advantages.

More recently, however, concern has been expressed in two main areas. The first concerns dependence, with possible cognitive impairment, particularly in long-term users. The second, more moral consideration is that of the medicalization of what are seen to be social problems or problems of living, and of encouraging, at least in the minds of the general public, the notion of 'a pill for every ill'.

In this Symposium, representatives of research and of clinicians who prescribe these drugs discussed the benefits and risks, their current use, the issue of long-term administration, the indications (such as they are), the place of benzodiazepines in general medicine and psychiatry, and the problem of unwanted side-effects.

Finally, an attempt was made to pull together the common themes that have emerged from the presentations and the discussions—members of the group debated the indications for the use of these drugs, what advice should be given about their use, and the clinical, pharmacological, and psychological contraindications, that is to say, guidelines concerning the use of one of the most popular drugs of the mid-1980s.

The benzodiazepines in current clinical practice, edited by Hugh Freeman and Yvonne Rue, 1987: Royal Society of Medicine Services International Congress and Symposium Series No. 114, published by Royal Society of Medicine Services Limited.

Benefits and risks of benzodiazepines

PETER TYRER

Mapperley Hospital, Nottingham NG3 6AA, UK

This account concentrates on the pharmacological benefits and risks of benzodiazepines that affect current clinical practice. It is a subject which can be looked at from a much wider perspective, including the cost-benefit analysis to society, but that aspect is discussed elsewhere in this volume (1). All effective treatments carry risks, and benzodiazepines are no exception; the ideal drug treatment does not exist, and if it did, the clinical skills of the practitioner — a subtle blend of observation, intuition and judgment — would not be needed. It is possible to argue that of these, judgment is the most important, and this involves a continuous balancing act in which benefits are weighed against risks in changing clinical situations. Because there are important differences between the benefits and risks of benzodiazepines in short- and long-term therapy, these will be discussed separately.

Short-term therapy

Benefits

Benzodiazepines are primarily used for the treatment of anxiety and insomnia, relief of muscle tension and spasticity, and as anticonvulsants. Their specific psychiatric and physical indications are dealt with in more detail by Professors Rickels and Turner in the present volume: for most it is important to have a rapid onset of clinical action, and sometimes desirable to have this within minutes. That can be achieved by the intravenous administration of benzodiazepines, which is used most often in anaesthetics and in the treatment of status epilepticus; intravenous diazepam is a well established and extremely valuable treatment for the latter condition (2). It is also sometimes necessary in psychiatric treatment to sedate violent and acutely disturbed patients safely and rapidly; benzodiazepines are highly suitable for this purpose, particularly when they are given intravenously. However, it is not always easy to give a drug by this route in such patients, and intramuscular injection may be the only alternative; in this situation, a rapidly absorbed preparation such as lorazepam may be highly beneficial (3,4).

The benzodiazepines in current clinical practice, edited by Hugh Freeman and Yvonne Rue, 1987: Royal Society of Medicine Services International Congress and Symposium Series No. 114, published by Royal Society of Medicine Services Limited.

When benzodiazepines are given by mouth the onset of action is more delayed, but clinical effects are normally shown within 45 min and are maximum within 2 h (5).

Benzodiazepines also have advantages in producing their clinical effects with a high safety margin and a relatively low incidence of acute adverse effects. This high specificity of clinical action is difficult to explain. There are specific binding sites in the central nervous system for benzodiazepines (6), and functional links between GABA receptors and benzodiazepine receptors (7). However, all the clinical actions of benzodiazepines are thought to be exerted by modulation of GABA transmission (8), as are the actions of other anti-anxiety drugs such as alcohol and the barbiturates, and no site specific for an anti-anxiety effect has yet been identified. It is possible that the therapeutic properties of drugs such as barbiturates and alcohol arise from their general membrane effects, which are not possessed by the benzodiazepines.

The benefits of benzodiazepines in short-term use become even more obvious when they are compared with other treatments for the relief of anxiety and other relevant conditions. Although alternative drugs such as the barbiturates may have a rapid onset of action, particularly when given intravenously, there is a much greater danger of severe cerebral depression, than with the benzodiazepines. For the relief of anxiety, benzodiazepines are superior in efficacy to barbiturates (9), and they have fewer hangover effects when given for insomnia (10).

Psychological methods of treating anxiety and insomnia, including cognitive therapy and anxiety management training, require several sessions of learning even by the most apt pupil, and are not useful in the treatment of short-term anxiety, unless the patient already has these skills. They are obviously not suitable either in the non-psychiatric indications for the benzodiazepines.

When measured against the benefits, the risks of benzodiazepines in short-term use are relatively small. In normal subjects studied under test conditions, benzodiazepines produce many effects on psychological functioning, including impairment of psychomotor performance and of central processing ability, particularly that concerned with sensory information (11). This can impair significantly the operating of machinery, tasks involving vigilance, and car driving ability (12). It is an important fact that those who take benzodiazepines are much more likely to have road accidents than those who do not (13), although it would be wrong to assume that the psychomotor effects of benzodiazepines are necessarily the cause of this.

Although this catalogue of adverse effects looks to be a serious one, the proper use of short-term benzodiazepines is at times of extreme stress and distress, and on such occasions it is unlikely that subjects would be carrying out complex psychomotor tasks. However, it has been known for many years (14) that in severe anxiety there is disintegration of performance in almost all areas of functioning, and in such patients benzodiazepines are likely in fact to lead to an improvement rather than a decrement in psychomotor functioning. It is also important that tolerance develops rapidly to these adverse effects, and that there is a progressive reduction in them after repeated use.

Anterograde amnesia may be both of benefit and a disadvantage: this is a well-established effect of benzodiazepines, that has been noted most frequently in anaesthetic practice (15). It only tends to be a prominent symptom at higher dosage, but may still be present with the therapeutic doses used for the treatment of anxiety. Although the induction of anterograde amnesia may be an advantage (e.g. in dental phobia), it can be a handicap in some stressful reactions, particularly those of great personal meaning that require acceptance before the conflict can be resolved. These include bereavements and other major losses, and memories of unpleasant events that tend to provoke the mental mechanism of denial; it seems likely that the

Table 1
Benefits and risks of benzodiazepines after short-term therapy (up to 2 weeks)

Benefits	Risks
Rapid onset of action	Interaction with central depressant drugs
High specificity	
Good safety margin	Impaired sensorimotor functioning
Low incidence of adverse effects	
More effective than other drugs	Anterograde amnesia

anterograde amnesic properties of benzodiazepines will promote such denial, and this could be counter-productive in the longer term (16).

When benzodiazepines are used for short-term indications, their benefits are great and far outweigh their risks (Table 1). They are well suited for the emergency treatment of adjustment and stress reactions and of disturbed behaviour in psychotic and violent patients. In these circumstances, the drug needs to be given for a maximum of two weeks, and significant improvement can often be seen after only a few doses. In such circumstances, the adverse effects of impaired sensorimotor performance and anterograde amnesia are relatively unimportant, although some care has to be taken if benzodiazepines are combined with other central depressant drugs (including alcohol) in view of the addictive effects. If benzodiazepines are used in this way, there is no risk of dependence, and they can be stopped without difficulty.

Long-term therapy

Benefits

A substantial proportion of those who take benzodiazepines take them on a long-term basis. The proportions vary between different countries (17) and have certainly fallen in the United States in recent years (18); however, it is still a matter of concern that approximately 20% of those taking benzodiazepines in the United States, and, if a recent MORI public opinion poll is to be believed, up to 35% in the United Kingdom, take them for four months or longer. The drugs are not recommended for this period of time (19), after which they are in any case no longer so effective (20).

Are there any benefits to patients who take benzodiazepines for at least six months, or in some cases for many years? Are there, in fact, any indications for permanent treatment with benzodiazepines? Taking all the evidence, there are few major hazards in taking benzodiazepines long-term; dosage tends to remain constant and there is no evidence of cumulative damage as, for example, in the case of alcohol. However, continued controversy has occurred over the interpretation of cognitive dysfunction in patients taking long-term benzodiazepines, and these issues are discussed by Professor Lader elsewhere in this volume.

When benzodiazepines are compared with other pharmacological agents for the long-term relief of anxiety, they do have advantages, but this does not mean that they confer benefit; it is only that 'damage limitation' is less with benzodiazepines than with barbiturates, alcohol, nicotine, and neuroleptic drugs. Clare (21) points out that since 'the implication is of a weary acceptance that psychotropics will always be with us, which poison appears to be most acceptable? But the choice, if there is to be a choice, is which is it to be—a cigarette, a drink, or a Valium?' He does not answer these questions directly, but there seems little doubt that a diazepam tablet is the least of the three evils.

When benzodiazepines are given specifically for their muscle relaxant and anti-convulsant effects, then long-term treatment is more appropriate. It is recognized that these conditions are often chronic, and sometimes permanent, so that long-term treatment is the rule. However, these indications form only a very small part of the total prescriptions for benzodiazepines.

Risks

The major hazard of long-term benzodiazepine consumption is dependence. This can be both psychological and physical, but in the last few years there has been increasing evidence that physical dependence is a much greater problem than was first suspected in the first 20 years of benzodiazepine use. There are several reasons for this delayed detection of a significant clinical problem. Among the most important of these is the fact that dependence rarely shows itself through increasing tolerance and escalation of dosage or through drug-seeking behaviour. It is manifest primarily by an abstinence syndrome after stopping the drug, which is immediately relieved by starting the drug again. There are many parallels between this type of dependence and cigarette smoking, as the level of consumption remains more or less the same, but temporarily increases at times of stress; drug consumption is maintained more through the symptoms of withdrawal than by the pleasurable effects of benzodiazepines (22).

Because psychological dependence is common with all anti-anxiety drugs, it is important for physical dependence to be demonstrated under double-blind conditions. This has been done unequivocally in several studies of patients withdrawn from benzodiazepines which had been taken for four months or longer in regular dosage (23,24,25). These and other studies have established that duration of treatment is an important factor in predisposing patients to the risk of dependence, but several additional factors, wholly or partly independent of long-term treatment, have also been established (Table 2).

There has been considerable controversy over the incidence of withdrawal syndromes in patients after stopping long-term benzodiazepines, as this ranges in different studies from 0% (30) to 100% (31). However, these differences can be explained largely by variation in the factors listed in Table 2. A population of anxious patients seen in primary care with adjustment difficulties to recognizable stresses is likely to have a very low incidence of withdrawal syndromes, whereas a selected psychiatric population who have tried repeatedly to reduce and stop their benzo-diazepines without success is likely to have a very high one.

As long-term therapy implies both regular dosage and some degree of psychological dependence, it is not surprising that withdrawal reactions are more common in this group. The suggestion that patients who have withdrawal reactions are more likely to have dependent personality characteristics carries face validity, but it is important to note that the measurement of these personality traits refers to premorbid or habitual function, and should therefore be independent of current pharmacological dependence.

The evidence that benzodiazepines with a short elimination (β) half-life are more likely to lead to withdrawal symptoms than those of longer half-life is disturbing, particularly for the pharmaceutical companies, who have attempted to refine the benzodiazepine drugs so that increasingly drugs of progressively shorter half-life are

Table 2
Factors increasing the risk of dependence with long-term use of benzodiazepines

Factor	Source
High dosage	Owen and Tyrer, 1983 (26)
Regular continuous dosage	Rickels et al., 1982 (20)
Previous drug dependence	Rickels et al., 1984 (27)
Dependent personality characteristics	Tyrer et al., 1983 (23)
High levels of psychological dependence	Murray, 1981 (28)
Benzodiazepines of short elimination half-life	Tyrer et al. 1981 (29)

being introduced to clinical practice. This reduces the incidence of hangover effects for hypnotic agents and may 'fine tune' the treatment of acute attacks of anxiety (including panic) so that the pharmacological actions are available when needed. However, if these apparently superior drugs are associated with a higher risk of dependence, their benefits disappear, and much more needs to be known about the differences in dependence risk between various benzodiazepines. These differences are unlikely to be explained completely by pharmacokinetic variations; the relative affinities of the drugs for the benzodiazepine receptors could be equally important (32).

Despite some extravagant claims that all patients who take long-term benzodiazepines become dependent, culminating recently in invitations to patients to sue practitioners who prescribe these drugs because of their dangers, a large proportion of patients stop taking benzodiazepines without any problems. When all the evidence is examined, the best estimate of dependence risk is that 60% of patients who stop benzodiazepines after several months' treatment will have no withdrawal symptoms (23,29). Of the remainder, approximately 10% return to their pre-existing anxiety levels, and 30% have a withdrawal syndrome.

This syndrome consists of well-known somatic and psychological symptoms of anxiety, particularly panic, insomnia, tremor, muscle tension, sweating, and palpitations (29,31,33,34) together with symptoms that are less prominent in anxiety states, including marked dysphoria (31), abnormal perceptual experiences (29,35), tinglings in hands and feet (36), and tinnitus (25). Unequivocal symptoms of physical dependence, including epileptic seizures (37), hallucinations, paranoid delusions, confusional states and the first-rank symptoms of schizophrenia (26,38,39), occur in less than 5% of all withdrawal reactions.

Although these symptoms, taken together, are indicative of a withdrawal syndrome, it is difficult to be certain in an individual patient whether the early symptoms are those of withdrawal or of a return to pre-existing anxiety. Many of these symptoms, including the perceptual ones, can be identified in normal subjects (40), and it is only the most serious (and least common) that are certainly those of physical dependence. Ashton (36) has also suggested that as some apparent withdrawal symptoms may become manifest during long-term treatment on regular dosage, this might indicate tolerance to the drug. This needs further enquiry; although tolerance does develop to the effects of benzodiazepines after periods up to seven weeks (41), most clinical experience suggests that this does not progress further.

The other major risk of long-term consumption of benzodiazepines, which is less apparent than symptoms of withdrawal and has attracted much less attention, is cognitive impairment; it is discussed by Professor Lader later in this book. Many of the symptoms of this impairment are subtle and difficult to detect, but they can be noted in retrospect by patients who have withdrawn from long-term treatment. Statements such as 'like walking in a fog' and 'losing control of my life' are used

Table 3
Benefits and risks of benzodiazepines after long-term therapy (more than 4 months)

Benefits	Risks
Good safety margin	Psychological dependence
Superior to most anti-anxiety drugs	Physical dependence
	Cognitive impairment

to describe the lack of initiative and ability to think clearly which occur when taking benzodiazepines persistently (42); the improvement in those following withdrawal is therefore a powerful reason for continuing with reducing programmes.

When the benefits and risks of long-term treatment are compared, the balance tilts against benefit. The lessened efficacy of long-term dosage, the increased risk of dependence, and the insidious cognitive effects can only be balanced against the relative safety of benzodiazepines compared with other anti-anxiety drug treatments (Table 3). However, even when compared with other drugs, benzodiazepines are no longer the preferred agents. There is now accumulated evidence that antidepressants are superior to benzodiazepines in relieving persistent anxiety symptoms (43,44,45), but this superiority usually requires several weeks of treatment before it is shown fully. It is independent of the presence of panic disorder (45) — a condition that is sometimes said to respond specifically to antidepressants — and also independent of depression. There is argument among nosologists about the status of anxiety as a diagnosis, but it is very difficult to argue that the anxious patients who respond to antidepressants do so because they are all fundamentally depressed.

Maximizing the benefits of benzodiazepines

Since benzodiazepines are so much more satisfactory as short-term treatments, is there any way of ensuring that they are used primarily for this purpose? All long-term consumers were originally short-term ones; what made them continue? There are several answers to these questions. Firstly, the universal recommendation that the benzodiazepines should be used for a few weeks only and then stopped (e.g. Committee on the Review of Medicines, 1980 (19)) is a little ingenuous, as it does not take into account either pressure from the patient to continue the prescription after this time, or the lack of an obvious alternative treatment. This pressure to continue may itself be indicative of a degree of pharmacological dependence. Kales et al. (46) introduced the term 'rebound insomnia' to describe a temporary increase in symptoms after stopping hypnotic benzodiazepines after a few weeks of treatment, and this phenomenon has been confirmed with most benzodiazepines of short or intermediate half-life. In general, the shorter the elimination half-life, the greater the withdrawal problems, which may explain some of the difficulties noted with the hypnotic benzodiazepine of shortest half-life—triazolam (47,48).

Similar 'rebound anxiety' has been found after benzodiazepines taken as tranquillizers are stopped after four to six weeks of regular treatment (49,50,51). Although the symptoms of these rebound phenomena are not as severe as some described in withdrawal syndromes, they show the typical time course of physical withdrawal symptoms, and are resolved by taking benzodiazepines again. It is therefore not surprising that many patients become distressed after their drugs are stopped and that they ask for continued prescription.

It is therefore possible to argue that most of the patients on long-term benzodiazepines become dependent soon after starting their drugs, and that continued prescription is determined more by withdrawal symptoms than by any other factor. However, although this hypothesis looks attractive, it cannot be sustained, as a large number of patients taking long-term benzodiazepines stop their drugs without any difficulty (23,29). Only a proportion become dependent, and it is best to try and identify these in advance.

Patients who are liable to become dependent tend to have recurrent anxiety in relationship to minor life events rather than major ones, and have dependent or obsessional personality characteristics. Their mood state varies, and anxiety and depression may be present at different times. This group is likely to take medication for a longer period and to respond better to tricyclic antidepressants (and to monoamine oxidase inhibitors) than to benzodiazepines (52). Benzodiazepines are more appropriately used for short-term anxiety that is likely to be self-limiting; such anxiety commonly follows major life events, and is common in adjustment reactions.

Careful prescribing can also reduce the risk of dependence. It is best to decide the period of benzodiazepine prescription in advance, to use intermittent flexible dosage wherever possible, and to reduce this gradually, even after short-term treatment (34,53).

All effective drugs carry dangers and need to be used judiciously. Benzodiazepines are no exception, but for many years have tended to be prescribed in a cavalier and sometimes irresponsible fashion. This has blighted their benefits and led to demands that they be banned (54). However, for many patients there is no satisfactory alternative to them at present, and, when used in the right way and for the right patient, they are effective, safe, and free of significant risk.

References

(1) Williams P. Long-term benzodiazepine use in general practice. In: Freeman HL and Rue Y, eds. *Benzodiazepines in current clinical practice.* Royal Society of Medicine International Congress and Symposium Series No. 114. London: Royal Society of Medicine 1987; 19–34.

(2) Parsonage MJ, Norris JW. Use of diazepam in treatment of severe convulsive status epilepticus. *Br Med J* 1967; **3**: 85–8.

(3) Bick PA, Hannah AL. Intramuscular lorazepam to restrain violent patients. *Lancet* 1986; **i**: 206.

(4) Jobling M, Stein G. Lorazepam in resistant mania. *Lancet* 1986; **i**: 510.

(5) Greenblatt DJ, Shader RI. *Benzodiazepines in clinical practice.* New York: Raven Press, 1974.

(6) Möhler H, Okada T. Benzodiazepine receptor: demonstration in the central nervous system. *Science* 1977; **198**: 849–51.

(7) Braestrup C, Nielsen M. Benzodiazepine receptors. *Arzneimittel-Forschung* 1980; **30**: 852–7.

(8) Haefely WE. Central actions of benzodiazepines: general introduction. *Br J Psych* 1978; **133**: 231–8.

(9) Lader MH, Bond AJ, James DC. Clinical comparison of anxiolytic drug therapy. *Psychol Med* 1974; **4**: 381–7.

(10) Bond AJ, Lader MH. Residual effects of hypnotics. *Psychopharmucologia* 1972; **25**: 117–32.

(11) Hindmarch I. Psychomotor function and psychoactive drugs. *Br J Clin Pharmacol* 1980; **10**: 189–210.

(12) Betts TA, Clayton AS, MacKay GM. Effects of four commonly used tranquillisers on low-speed driving performance tests. *Br Med J* 1972; **288**: 1135–40.

(13) Skegg DCG, Richards SM, Doll R. Minor tranquillisers and road accidents. *Br Med J* 1979; **1**: 917-9.
(14) Yerkes RM, Dodson JD. The relation of strength of stimulus to rapidity of habit-formation. *J Comp Neurol Psychol* 1908; **18**: 459-82.
(15) Dundee JW, Pandit SK. Anterograde amnesic effects of pethidine, hyoscine and diazepam in adults. *Br J Pharmacol* 1972; **44**: 140-4.
(16) Tyrer P. The place of tranquillisers in the management of stress. *J Psychosom Res* 1983; **27**: 385-90.
(17) Balter MB, Levine J, Manheimer DI. Cross-national study of the extent of antianxiety/sedative drug use. *New Engl J Med* 1974; **29**: 769-74.
(18) Mellinger GD, Balter MB. Prevalence and patterns of use of psychotherapeutic drugs: results from a 1979 national survey of American adults. In: Tosnoni G, Bellantuono C, Lader M, eds. *Epidemiological impacts of psychotropic drugs*. Amsterdam: Elsevier/North Holland, 1981: 117-35.
(19) Committee on the Review of Medicines. Systematic review of the benzodiazepines. *Br Med J* 1980; **280**: 910-12.
(20) Rickels K, Case WG, Downing RW. Issues in long-term treatment with benzodiazepines. *Psychopharmacol Bull* 1982; **18**: 38-41.
(21) Clare AW. Benzodiazepines, alcohol or nicotine? In: Trimble MR, ed. *Benzodiazepines divided*. Chichester: John Wiley & Sons, 1983: 1-14.
(22) Murphy SM, Tyrer P. The essence of benzodiazepine dependence. *Br J Addiction* 1987: (in press).
(23) Tyrer P, Owen R, Dawling S. Gradual withdrawal of diazepam after long-term therapy. *Lancet* 1981; **ii**: 520-22.
(24) Petursson H, Lader M. *Dependence on tranquillisers*. London: Oxford University Press, 1984.
(25) Busto U, Sellers E, Naranjo CA, Cappell H, Sanchez-Craig M, Sykora K. Withdrawal reaction after long-term therapeutic use of benzodiazepines. *New Engl J Med* 1986; **315**: 854-9.
(26) Owen RT, Tyrer P. Benzodiazepine dependence: a review of the evidence. *Drugs* 1983; **25**: 385-98.
(27) Rickels K, Case WG, Winokur A, Swenson C. Long-term benzodiazepine therapy: benefits and risks. *Psychopharmacol Bull* 1984; **20**: 608-15.
(28) Murray J. Long-term psychotropic drug-taking and the process of withdrawal. *Psychol Med* 1981; **11**: 853-8.
(29) Tyrer P, Rutherford D, Huggett T. Benzodiazepine withdrawal symptoms and propranolol. *Lancet* 1981; **ii**: 520-522.
(30) Bowden CL, Fisher JG. Safety and efficacy of long-term benzodiazepine therapy. *South Med J* 1980; **73**: 1581-4.
(31) Petursson H, Lader MH. Withdrawal from long-term benzodiazepine treatment. *Br Med J* 1981; **283**: 643-5.
(32) Lancet. Editorial. Treatment of benzodiazepine dependence. *Lancet* 1987; **i**: 78-9.
(33) Covi L, Lipman RS, Pattison JH, Derogatis LR, Uhlenhuth EH. Length of treatment with anxiolytic sedatives and response to their sudden withdrawal. *Acta Psych Scand* 1983; **49**: 51-64.
(34) Tyrer P, Seivewright N. Use of beta blocker drugs in withdrawal states. *Postgrad Med J* 1984; **60**: 47-50.
(35) Schopf J. Unusual withdrawal symptoms after long-term administration of benzodiazepines. *Nervenarzt* 1981; **52**: 288-92.
(36) Ashton H. Benzodiazepine withdrawal: an unfinished story. *Br Med J* 1984; **288**: 1135-40.
(37) Howe JG. Lorazepam withdrawal seizures. *Br Med J* 1980; **280**: 1164-4.
(38) Tan T-L, Bixler EO, Kales A, Cadieux RJ, Goodman AL. Early morning insomnia, daytime anxiety and organic mental disorder associated with triazolam. *J Fam Pract* 1985; **20**: 592-4.
(39) Roberts K, Case WG, Winokur A, Swenson C. Long-term benzodiazepine therapy: benefits and risks. *Psychopharmacol Bull* 1984; **20**: 608-15.

(40) Rodrigo EK, Williams P. Frequency of self-reported 'anxiolytic withdrawal' symptoms in a group of female students experiencing anxiety. *Psychol Med* 1986; **16**: 467–72.
(41) Kales A, Bixler EO, Soldatos CR, Vela-Bueno A, Jacoby J, Kales JD. Quazepam and flurazepam: long-term use and extended withdrawal. *Clin Pharmacol Ther* 1982; **32**: 781–8.
(42) Tyrer P. *How to stop taking tranquillisers.* London: Sheldon Press, 1986.
(43) Johnstone EC, Owens DG, Frith CD, McPherson K, Dowie C, Riley G, Gold A. Neurotic illness and its response to anxiolytic and antidepressant treatment. *Psychol Med* 1980 **10**: 321–8.
(44) McNair DM, Kahn RJ. Imipramine compared with a benzodiazepine for agoraphobia. In: Klein DF, Rabkin JG, eds. *Anxiety: new research and changing concepts.* New York: Raven Press, 1981: 69–80.
(45) Kahn RJ, McNair DM, Lipman RS *et al.* Imipramine and chlordiazepoxide in depressive and anxiety disorders: 2: Efficacy in anxious out-patients. *Arch Gen Pysch* 1986; **43**: 79–85.
(46) Kales A, Scharf MB, Kales JD. Rebound insomnia: a new clinical syndrome. *Science* 1978; **201**: 1039–41.
(47) Van der Kroef C. Reactions to triazolam. *Lancet* 1979; **ii**: 256.
(48) Griffiths RR, Lamb RJ, Ator NA, Roache JD, Brady JV. Relative abuse liability of triazolam: experimental assessment in animals and humans. *Neurosci Biobehav Rev* 1985; **9**: 133–51.
(49) Fontaine R, Chouinard G, Annable L. Rebound anxiety in anxious patients after abrupt withdrawal of benzodiazepine treatment. *Am J Psych* 1984; **141**: 848–52.
(50) Murphy SM, Owen RT, Tyrer PJ. Withdrawal symptoms after six weeks treatment with diazepam. *Lancet* 1984; **ii**: 1389.
(51) Power KG, Jerrom DWA, Simpson RJ, Mitchell M. Controlled study of withdrawal symptoms and rebound anxiety after six week course of diazepam for generalised anxiety. *Br Med J* 1985; **290**: 1246–8.
(52) Tyrer P. Neurosis divisible. *Lancet* 1985; **i**: 685–8.
(53) Lader MH, Higgitt AC. Management of benzodiazepine dependence—update 1986. *Br J Addiction* 1986; **81**: 7–10.
(54) Snaith RP. Benzodiazepines on trial. *Br Med J* 1984; **288**: 1379.

Discussion

Professor Lader took exception to the view that the benzodiazepines were specific anxiolytics; their biochemical action was such that they could not be so and there was no evidence of special anxiety-mediating mechanisms in the brain which were affected by them. The fact that certain high-affinity receptors existed did not make the drug's action specific. If that was not borne in mind, there was a danger of playing down the problems of these drugs, which largely arose because they were non-specific. If they really were specific, they would be purely anxiolytic, so that there would then be no side-effects, and no problems of dependence. However, **Dr Tyrer** suggested that their safety depended partly on their *relative* specificity, compared with other compounds.

Dr File pointed out that a specific binding site did not make the drug's action specific, nor did it make the drug safer. The fact that it was a modulatory site rather than a neurotransmitter site might make for greater safety, (and so the nature of the site rather than its existence might be important), but as the barbiturates also bound to a specific site on the same complex, that argument was dubious.

Professor Rickels had found no drug yet which had better anxiolytic properties than the benzodiazepines. All drugs have a number of actions, but until a specific anxiolytic with no side-effects becomes available, the benzodiazepines are the most useful for the treatment of anxiety.

Dr File said that was not in question, it was the mechanism of action that was under discussion.

Professor Clare was a little puzzled as to the sudden emphasis on specificity, since he found it difficult to think of any highly specific drug with specific actions.

Mr Taylor said that there could presumably be a more specific drug in Professor Lader's terms, which would have undesirable side effects.

Professor Lader agreed but said that nevertheless, continuing to believe that benzodiazepines were specific would lead to problems.

Dr Beary referred to research at St George's Hospital on the risk of benzodiazepine abuse. Amongst drug addicts attending the St George's Clinic for three months in 1984 and 1985, 60% had benzodiazepines in their urine. Although these drugs were taken for abuse purposes, prescriptions for them were obtained from general practitioners. On the black market, a pill such as 10 mg Valium™ sold for about 10p.

Current usage of benzodiazepines in Britain

DAVID TAYLOR

The Association of the British Pharmaceutical Industry, Whitehall, London SW1A 2DY, UK

This paper presents statistical data relating to the consumption of benzodiazepine-containing medicine in Great Britain; social aspects of the debate relating to benzodiazepine dependence are discussed, as well as economic issues relating to benzodiazepine supply. It is suggested that the significance of direct charges to patients in helping to ensure appropriate consumption of tranquillizer/sedative medicine may have been unduly neglected.

Consumption statistics

Benzodiazepine-containing medicines first became available in the UK at the start of the 1960s, when the hypnotic/tranquillizer market was dominated by relatively hazardous barbiturate products. The search for safer alternatives to the latter received a significant setback in the form of the thalidomide tragedy. But from 1965 onwards barbiturate usage began to decline in Britain, while that of benzodiazepine medicines increased rapidly. In 1960, there were some 27–28 million Family Practitioner Service (FPS) prescription items dispensed which were classified either as hypnotics or tranquillizers, of which over 15 million were barbiturate hypnotics. By 1974, this total had risen to about 40 million items, of which just under 25 million were benzodiazepines and around 8 million barbiturate hypnotics. Although it is impossible to make fully accurate comparisons on the basis of prescription item numbers, this is evidence of a significant relative increase (circa 40%) in psychotropic medicine usage. However, over the same period, alcohol consumption in the United Kingdom rose from approximately 4·5 litres of absolute alcohol per capita per annum to 7·5 litres—a 66% growth.

Examination of more detailed DHSS data relating to the period 1974–1985 shows that the total number of benzodiazepine-containing prescription items dispensed by the FPS (Great Britain) rose from 24·6 million in the former year to a peak of almost 31 million in 1979: by 1985, it had fallen back to an estimated 26 million—a 16% decline in 6 years. (There may, however, have been a very modest rise in private prescriptions dispensed in this last year.)

The benzodiazepines in current clinical practice, edited by Hugh Freeman and Yvonne Rue, 1987: Royal Society of Medicine Services International Congress and Symposium Series No. 114, published by Royal Society of Medicine Services Limited.

When prescriptions for benzodiazepine hypnotics are separated from those classed as tranquillizers, two quite different patterns emerge. FPS-dispensed benzodiazepine hypnotic items rose in number steadily throughout the 1970s, from under 5 million at the start of that decade to 13 million at the commencement of the 1980s; the 1985 estimated total stood at some 14 million items. By contrast, the number of benzodiazepine tranquillizer prescriptions which were dispensed increased from about 10 million in 1970 to a peak of 18 million in 1978. The 1985 estimated total was 12 million items—one third down on the figure of seven years previously.

Looking at benzodiazepine usage by substance, the number of prescription items dispensed containing diazepam, nitrazepam, or chlordiazepoxide fell by 12·5 million between 1978 and 1985. By contrast, those for temazepam and lorazepam increased by 5·5 million; these trends together represent a significant shift in the balance of usage towards products with a shorter plasma half-life.

Finally, in the context of basic consumption statistics, the most significant consumer variables associated with prescribing of benzodiazepines are sex and age. World-wide, female consumption rates are about twice those of males, and it may be estimated that some 40–45% of benzodiazepine prescription items dispensed in the UK via the FPS are supplied to patients aged over 65.

If tranquillizers and hypnotics are separated, then the age relationship still holds constant in Britain; in both cases, about 70% of both benzodiazepine hypnotics and tranquillizers are dispensed to females. But the age breakdowns differ: in the case of tranquillizers, female consumption rates in all age-groups over 40 are high, and roughly equal. It is estimated that the 13 million British women aged over 40 receive almost 60% of all the benzodiazepine medicines prescribed for the UK population. But in the context of hypnotics, there is a more even increase in consumption with age: the five million British women aged over 65 probably consume around 40% of all benzodiazepine hypnotics supplied via the FPS, whereas the eight million aged between 40 and 65 take about 25% of the national total.

These figures are in large part a mirror-image of those relating to alcohol consumption. Data relating to the late 1970s indicate that among those British males who drink regularly (as do 75–80%) those in their twenties admit to consuming the equivalent of around 13 pints of beer a week: thise is more than twice the level of intake reported by males past retirement age. Of the 50–60% of women who take alcohol weekly, those in their 60s or over report an intake equivalent to 2½ pints every 7 days—half that of women in their twenties.

Long-term usage and benzodiazepine dependence

The available data do not make it possible to estimate with accuracy the extent of long-term benzodiazepine usage in the community, or the numbers at risk of experiencing distressing withdrawal symptoms, were they suddenly to discontinue their medication. However, it may be estimated that about three benzodiazepine tranquillizer prescriptions in every four are repeats, and that for hypnotics, the ratio is probably five out of six. Linking these observations to a number of other published estimates of the extent of overall and long-term benzodiazepine usage in the population, the following rough estimates for Britain can be derived:

    Number of consumers taking benzodiazepines on a
      short-term basis in each year (up to and around three months)   c.3 million
    Number of consumers taking benzodiazepines on a
      medium-term basis in each year (around six months)   c.500 000

Number of consumers taking benzodiazepines on a
long-term basis (a year or more)   c.1·2 million
(Based on Balter *et al.* (1)—a 1981 survey.)

It should be noted, however, that these crude estimates may not adequately take into account the fact that perhaps 10% of benzodiazepines are prescribed for non-psychiatric indications and that some 'regular' long-term users may in practice take their medicines on an 'as needed' rather than a day-to-day basis. There is inevitably a significant amount of wastage, with unwanted medicines being discarded, and it appears that dispensing levels have reduced significantly in the last few years.

Taken together, such considerations mean that the total numbers of regular medium- and long-term users could well now be significantly below the estimates shown above, and that it would be rash to hazard any firm guess as to the numbers of individuals who may currently be said to be benzodiazepine-dependent and/or at significant risk of unpleasant withdrawal symptoms. Future studies might usefully differentiate more precisely between daytime and 'tranquillizer' usage of benzodiazepines, and their employment as hypnotics. The long-term use of such medication in the elderly (65+) population is also a subject worthy of particular attention.

On occasions, the hazard to society presented by benzodiazepine dependence has been exaggerated (2). The reasons for this range from 'pharmacological puritanism' to the fact that the issues surrounding benzodiazepine usage fulfil many of the criteria necessary for the creation of commercially profitable news/publishing 'stories'. Nevertheless, unnecessary usage of medicines of any type is to be discouraged, especially as a minority of consumers may experience distress as a result of excessive, ill-advised benzodiazepine use. Prescribers and producers alike may be accused of neglect if they fail to examine the costs and benefits of all forms of medicine usage as vigorously as possible.

Economic aspects

In respect of the economic aspects of benzodiazepine usage in Great Britain, there are three main points. The first is the apparent cheapness of benzodiazepine therapy (net ingredient cost under £2 per prescription) compared with alternatives such as individual patient counselling: the second is linked to the recent (1985) introduction of the NHS limited list, which has mainly affected medicines available 'over-the-counter', but which among prescription products has particularly involved benzodiazepines: and the third is based on data which suggest that extended patient charges might significantly influence benzodiazepine usage.

In the early 1980s, benzodiazepine-containing medicines accounted for a total NHS outlay of around £50 million (hospital and community), whereas total consumer spending on alcohol in the UK was over £13 billion in 1983. Thus, benzodiazepines represented some 3% of the total NHS medicine costs (in manufacturer's prices) and 0·3% of all NHS spending, yet they were contained in 8% of all the prescription items dispensed by the FPS. They were therefore 'cheap' even before the introduction of the limited list in terms of average medicine costs, and also relative to other health service inputs (medical and equivalent professional labour costs around £15/h). This factor, rather than some hypothesized draining of health service resources due to benzodiazepine purchases, may lie at the bottom of any failure of the NHS to provide alternative/complementary provisions, such as general practice-based psychological counselling for 'neurotically' distressed patients.

In the context of the limited list, the benzodiazepines represented a politically vulnerable target, in a situation in which there was great pressure to reduce the cost of medicines. The impact of the list has been to cut total NHS benzodiazepine outlays by around 20% in its first year of operation. This may be seen as desirable, although it also served to cut some British jobs and pharmaceutical industry investment. It may also in future permit relatively unopposed entry to the market place for new non-benzodiazepine anxiolytics, unless controls are extended to cover other categories of psychotropic product. Yet any such move would be undesirable, in as much as it might disrupt therapeutic progress, and further discourage research.

In conclusion, DHSS data on the impact of raised prescription charges on the consumption of tranquillizers (all types) in the period 1976-1983 should also be considered. There was a 50% fall between 1979 and 1983 in chargeable tranquillizer prescriptions dispensed. It was in 1979 that charge increases were imposed for the first time in several years. By contrast, the number of charge-exempt tranquillizers prescriptions rose slightly between 1979 and 1983. Data such as these could have encouraged Ministers to fear that unnecessary benzodiazepine consumption was occurring in the exempted population in the early 1980s. Despite trends such as the growing number of elderly consumers and rising unemployment (increasing the numbers of distressed, charge-exempt patients), the divergence between the trends for dispensing (as opposed to writing) exempt and non-exempt tranquillizer prescriptions in the period described is striking. It raises the possibility that if reduced benzodiazepine consumption is really seen as a desirable social goal, the number of people entitled to charge-free prescriptions should be decreased.

There would be equity problems to be resolved were such a proposal seriously to be considered, but some form of special exemption for all those clearly in need of free anxiolytic/sedative medication could probably be introduced.

Increased direct prices are an effective way to moderate alcohol consumption, and it may be argued that in several key respects people are, or should be, as much in control of their own use of benzodiazepines as they are in the case of alcohol. However, political factors could well discourage those in authority from examining closely this option—which partly explains why the NHS limited list of medicines was brought into being.

A medical comment

by Frank Wells

This subject is one with which I was closely associated in my days in clinical practice, prior to 1979—specifically the control of the misuse of drugs, and within that context, of amphetamines and barbiturates. Regarding amphetamines, a corporate policy taken by all prescribing doctors in a given geographical district not to prescribe a specific substance, and by all pharmacists not to stock it, led to the virtual elimination of a drug with potential for abuse for over a decade (3). Experience gained from this exercise enabled a similar policy to be adopted for barbiturates, on this occasion using an alternative group of drugs—the benzodiazepines—as a transitory expedient (4,5). It was better understanding of amphetamines and barbiturates by doctors which led to their being more responsibly prescribed, and the same process should occur in the case of benzodiazepines. However, it would be quite wrong to compare the usefulness of benzodiazepines with that of barbiturates, given the very considerable difference in risk/benefit ratio between the two.

There is already a reduction, for whatever reason, in the overall prescribing of benzodiazepine tranquillizers as David Taylor has pointed out. On the other hand, a similar fall in the prescribing of benzodiazepine hypnotics has not so far occurred, and we are still seeing some degree of dependence on them in the general community. This could be self-limiting, but nevertheless exists at present. However, I believe the problem is exaggerated, particularly in the media, and that the hazards are nothing like those of barbiturate dependence with which many doctors were previously familiar. Nor did I find in general practice that the treatment of benzodiazepine dependence presented the same degree of challenge found with that for barbiturates. Although there had been many such patients, when I left my practice in 1979, I had none on such drugs for longer than four months (6). For short-term and for intermittent hypnotic use, they were prescribed as appropriate, and are still excellent.

The pharmaceutical industry strives to have a responsible attitude towards the use of the drugs it manufactures. It would be quite counter-productive if it was thought to be promoting or even associated with the irresponsible use of its own products.

I would like to see the misuse of benzodiazepines minimized in clinical practice, so that they are perceived as being highly effective, relatively safe, and extremely useful members of the armamentarium with which doctors are familiar.

References

(1) Balter MH, Manheimer DI, Melinger GD, Uhlenhuth EH. A cross-national comparison of antianxiety/sedative drug use. *Curr Med Res Opinion* 1984; **8**: 5-20.
(2) Bury MR, Gabe J. 1987 (in press).
(3) Wells FO. The effects of a voluntary ban on amphetamine prescribing by doctors on abuse patterns—experience in the United Kingdom. In: *Amphetamine and related stimulants*. Oxford: Blackwell, 1975: 189-92.
(4) Wells FO. Prescribing barbiturates: drug substitution in general practice. *J Roy Coll Gen Pract* 1973; **25**: 164-7.
(5) Wells FO. Drug dependence in general practice. *Gen Pract Int* 1977; **4**: 176-9.
(6) Wells FO. The end of the barbiturate era. *Sleep Topics* 1981; **2**: 3-8.

Discussion

Professor Clare, referring to Dr Wells' statement that a better understanding of the amphetamines and barbiturates by doctors led to a reduction in misuse, said he had understood that what actually produced an alteration in prescribing was rather the development of better drugs. In the case of amphetamines it was the introduction of antidepressants, and in the case of barbiturates, that of the benzodiazepines.

Dr Wells said that a better understanding by doctors of the dependence potential of a drug had prevented them allowing patients to continue on it for a longer period than was clinically necessary, and also enabled them to ensure that patients were weaned off the drug or treated for the dependence.

Dr Imlah pointed out that there was more amphetamine misuse today than at the height of prescribing of amphetamines; after alcohol, amphetamines were probably the most abused drug in the country. Whether as a result of a campaign against the prescribing of amphetamines or other factors, one outcome had been an actual increase in the amount of amphetamine abuse.

Professor Turner thought that one of the reasons why the Curb Campaign (Campaign to Urge the Restriction of Barbiturates and other tranquillizers) had been so successful was that there was an alternative to barbiturates available, in the form of the benzodiazepines. This was not the case for the other drugs of dependence.

Dr Marks asked whether, in view of the divergence between charged and exempt prescriptions, there would be any support for the removal of the benzodiazepines from their prescription-only status.

Dr Wells thought that the majority of those concerned professionally would not think it appropriate to take benzodiazepines off prescription; certainly, the pharmaceutical industry would not wish to do so.

Mr Taylor strongly agreed and raised the issue of the Limited List. The consequences of removing exemptions from charges on elderly people were politically non-viable, regardless of the welfare argument; Treasury pressure around 1984 to make savings in the health budget had therefore resulted in the limited list.

Dr File pointed out that not only were drugs paid for, but also alcohol: there was so much cross-dependence between the two that the accounting process should compare the cost, e.g. of a bottle of sherry with that of a container of diazepam.

Dr Higgs believed that elderly people paid for their drugs in more than money terms, and that a distinction should be made between tranquillizers and hypnotics. Most prescriptions for the elderly were for sleep problems, and it was difficult to predict the consequences if a large number of people decided to put themselves to sleep by other methods.

Professor Turner pointed out that an over-the counter hypnotic, promethazine, was sold in pharmacies, and it had been suggested that a benzodiazepine should be similarly available.

Professor Lader said that where benzodiazepines had been freely available, as in certain countries in the Third World, it had been a public health disaster: there had been a tremendous amount of chronic abuse, and in almost all cases the Authorities had eventually moved to put the benzodiazepines onto a prescription-only basis. An antihistamine was a different matter, because those compounds did not have the associated dangers.

Dr Tyrer said that the principle of removing prescription controls was not only relevant to promethazine, but also to vodka: if vodka was in front of the Committee for the Safety of Medicine as a new drug, it would not be approved for any purpose. However, to say that because one evil was condoned a second evil should be condoned was not acceptable.

Dr Marks said that if the restraints on alcohol introduced during World War I were restored, the problem of alcohol abuse might be reduced, and it was likely that benzodiazepines could also be controlled by fiscal measures.

Mr Taylor thought that the partnership between patient and doctor in understanding and identifying the problem was one factor, and that the direct cash cost to the patient was another, but they were not mutually exclusive. He agreed that there was a time-and-effort cost for elderly patients, which was not experienced in the same way as a cash cost. As to the relationship between alcohol and benzodiazepines, there was almost a mirror image between the high use in elderly women of benzodiazepines, and the high use of alcohol in young men.

Professor Clare thought that societal structure was such that men were encouraged to go to the pub and off-licence, while women were encouraged to go to the general practitioner.

Long-term benzodiazepine use in general practice

PAUL WILLIAMS

*General Practice Research Unit, Institute of Psychiatry,
De Crespigny Park, London SE5 8AF*

The large and regular increases in the number of prescriptions for benzodiazepines and other psychotropic drugs that occurred during the late 1960s and early 1970s are well-known and frequently commented on (1,2,3). However, the significance of such trends in prescribing, in relation to trends in long-term use, is not clear, since such data are based on counts of prescriptions and not of people. Thus, increases in prescriptions could reflect an increase in the number of consumers as a whole, an increase in the number of prescriptions per consumer (whether due to increasing long-term use or to decreasing amounts of drug per prescription), an increase in the amount of drugs prescribed but not consumed, or any combination of these factors.

In order to investigate this, Williams (4) compared population- and general practice-based surveys of the extent of psychotropic drugs prescription and consumption (Table 1). Comparison of two large-scale studies of prescribing by general practitioners in England suggests that the increases in prescribing that occurred in the late 1960s and early 1970s were accompanied by an increase in the proportion of the population receiving a prescription for a psychotropic drug. However, comparison of three population surveys of consumption of psychotropic drugs indicates that there was no comparable increase in the proportion of the population who reported consuming such drugs; (these comparisons are predicated on the assumption that such sets of surveys can be compared—see Murray *et al.* (7) and Williams (4) for evidence to support this assumption). Williams (4) noted that this disparity (between prescribing and consuming) could be explained in a number of ways; but there was evidence to suggest that the most likely was in terms of a decrease in compliance and an increase in long-term drug use. This interpretation is supported by Marks' demonstration of substantial increases in the extent to which benzodiazepines are prescribed on a 'repeat' basis (9).

Since the mid-1970s there has been a levelling off and a subsequent decrease in the prescribing of benzodiazepines and other tranquillizers (10)—a pattern which has been found in most countries for which data are available (but not all—Italy is an exception (11)). The prime factor in this decrease is most likely to have been a reduction in new prescribing (i.e. a decreasing rate of incident benzodiazepine use) rather than wholesale discontinuation of treatment by long-term consumers. This suggests that

---

The benzodiazepines in current clinical practice, edited by Hugh Freeman and Yvonne Rue, 1987: Royal Society of Medicine Services International Congress and Symposium Series No. 114, published by Royal Society of Medicine Services Limited.

Table 1
The extent of psychotropic drug use in England

	No, place, year of study	Rate (%)
One year prevalence of prescribing		
Parish (1)	13259 Birmingham 1969	12·6
Skegg et al. (5)	36280 Oxfordshire 1974	19·3[a]
Two-week prevalence of consumption		
Dunnell & Cartwright (6)	1412 England 1969	11·0
Murray et al. (7)	5833 West London 1977	10·9
Anderson (8)	836 England 1977	12·0

[a]Of those aged >15 years

there is a cohort of long-term benzodiazepine users, created during the phase of enthusiasm in the mid-1960s and early 1970s, from which members will slowly be lost (a small proportion will discontinue treatment, others will die) and to which few new members will be recruited, since a reduction in new prescribing will inevitably lead to fewer people becoming long-term users (however 'long-term' is defined).

Factors relating to long-term use

From the research point of view, one response to these trends in benzodiazepine use and to the concern which they engendered, both lay and professional (12), has been to search for factors which are related to long-term drug prescription and consumption. Such factors may be interpreted in two ways. Firstly, they may be considered as predisposing to long-term use: such an interpretation is most appropriate at a time when the prime concern is about the increasing extent of long-term use. Alternatively, they may be regarded as factors which militate against discontinuation of treatment—an interpretation more useful if there is indeed a relatively static cohort of long-term users.

A number of retrospective and cross-sectional studies have examined this topic, but in the main, the emphasis has been on demographic and clinical aspects of long-term users of benzodiazepines and other psychotropic drugs, while social features have been relatively neglected.

Demographic factors

There is general agreement that sex and age are related to prolonged psychotropic drug use. For example, Woodcock (13) carried out a retrospective analysis of the medical records of 20 general practitioners to identify patients who had received 'a daily dosage of a psychotropic drugs for at least one year'; four-fifths of these were aged 40 years or more, and three-quarters were women. Similarly, Parish (1), in his retrospective case-note survey of the work of 48 general practitioners in Birmingham, found that when he studied patients who had received psychotropic drugs continuously for one year or more, 'the ratio of female to male patients was higher than for the overall sex ratio of all patients on psychotropic drug therapy . . . (and) . . . those patients on prolonged therapy tended to be ten years older than the patients on psychotropic drug therapy in general'.

These studies were carried out when barbiturates constituted the predominant category of psychotropic drug, but while the drugs may have changed, the findings have not. For example, Cooperstock (14,15), in her cross-sectional studies in Canada, found that women were more likely than men to receive multiple prescriptions for minor tranquillizers and other psychotropic drugs, while Mellinger et al.'s (16) population survey in the United States found that long-term regular users of anxiolytics tend to be older persons . . . (and) . . . are predominantly women'. Similar findings emerged from our recent study (17). We identified all patients who had received prescriptions for benzodiazepines continuously for one year or more in one south London general practice; 82 such patients were identified, constituting $2 \cdot 2\%$ of the practice list, and 64 agreed to be interviewed. The median duration of treatment was just over 5 years, with a range of 1–25 years; 48 of the patients (75%) were female and 40 (63%) were aged 60 years or more.

Clinical aspects

There is evidence that long-term users of benzodiazepines and other tranquillizers experience high levels of emotional distress. Mellinger et al. (16) described 68 respondents from a community survey who reported regular (daily for one year or more) use of anxiolytics. They found that half of these long-term users had high scores on their questionnaire measure of emotional distress—the PSYDIS (18)—as compared with 20% of the non-users, but noted that in this respect, 'the long-term users did not differ much from the other users', 45% of whom were high scorers.

In our study of long-term benzodiazepine users in general practice (17), we found that 22 (34%) of the 64 patients interviewed were rated by the interviewing psychiatrists as cases on the Standardised Psychiatric Interview (19)—a semi-structured interview designed to quantify psychiatric disorder in non-psychiatric settings. While in absolute terms this is a substantial level of psychiatric morbidity, it is not very different from that which would be found in an unselected series of general practice attenders. For example, Marks et al. (20) obtained a case rate of 39% in their study of patients attending 91 general practitioners in Manchester, while Skuse and Williams (21) recorded a level of 34% in a south London general practice; in both cases, the Standardised Psychiatric Interview was used as the case criterion.

The interviewing psychiatrists in our study of long-term benzodiazepine users also assigned an ICD diagnosis to the 22 patients classified as cases: 19 of them were allotted an ICD diagnosis relating to depression (ICD nos. $296 \cdot 1$, $300 \cdot 4$ and $309 \cdot 0$), but only one patient was allotted an anxiety-related diagnosis (ICD $300 \cdot 2$). While this was in some ways an unexpected finding, there is evidence that the use of tranquillizers is widespread in the treatment of depressed persons in the community. For example, Weissman and Klerman (22) followed-up 150 depressed women who had responded to tricyclic antidepressants and who had received 8 months of maintenance treatment as part of a controlled clinical trial. When followed-up one and four years after the maintenance treatment had ended, these women were more likely to receive a minor tranquillizer than an antidepressant when they sought medical help. Furthermore, when Gullick and King (23) studied patients attending a marital and sexual counselling centre, they noted that those with major depressive disorders were more likely to have received a minor tranquillizer than an antidepressant. Similar findings were obtained by Weissman *et al.* (24) in their community survey of depression and its treatment in the United States.

There is evidence that *de novo* prescription of benzodiazepines and other psychotropic drugs frequently occurs in response to physical rather than psychological disorder (25,26), so that it is not surprising that this has been investigated in the context of long-term drug use. Murray *et al.* (27) interviewed 22 patients who had been prescribed psychotropic drugs continuously for six months or more; they found that 'chronic physical complaints were common in the sample (diverticulitis, arthritis, hypertension, migraine) and 13 people were long-term users of non-psychotropic prescribed drugs'. Furthermore, in a questionnaire study of present and past long-term tranquillizer users (28) only 6 out of 261 respondents scored as having no disability or physical symptoms on the Belloc scale (29).

Mellinger *et al.* (16), in the study of 68 long-term consumers of anxiolytics referred to above, found that physical health distinguished between long-term users and other users more sharply than did any other factor they studied (including emotional distress). They noted that 'at least one-third of the long-term users reported four or more health problems—a rate twice that found among the other anxiolytic users and seven times that of the non users'. These differences persisted when age was controlled for, and they observed further that much of the difference between the long-term users and the others could be accounted for by cardiovascular disorders and arthritis.

Our study in south London (17) confirmed Mellinger *et al.*'s findings in that the patients reported substantial physical morbidity. For example, 27 (42%) had consulted their GP during the previous month for a physical illness (other than coughs, colds and influenza), and 22 (34%) had attended medical or surgical outpatient clinics in the previous year.

Prospective studies of long-term use

So far, the studies referred to have been retrospective or cross-sectional investigations of individuals identified as long-term users of benzodiazepines and other psychotropic durgs. However, we conducted a longitudinal prospective study of psychotropic drug use in a general practice setting (27,30,31) and to our knowledge, it is the only investigation in which this strategy has been used. Six general practitioners in south London were asked to identify and provide information about those patients to whom they supplied a new prescription for a psychotropic drug. 'New' was defined so as to include first-ever prescriptions as well as those written for the treatment of a new episode of illness; subsequent prescribing was monitored for six months.

One-hundred-and-fifty-four patients were entered into the study, and follow-up prescribing information was available for 124 (81%) of these. For each patient, the duration of continuous treatment was calculated, defined according to the method of Parish (1) as the length of time elapsing between the initiation of treatment and the day on which medication would have been used up if it had been taken according to prescription (this is of course not necessarily the same as duration of consumption). Survival curves were then plotted, using these duration of treatment data.

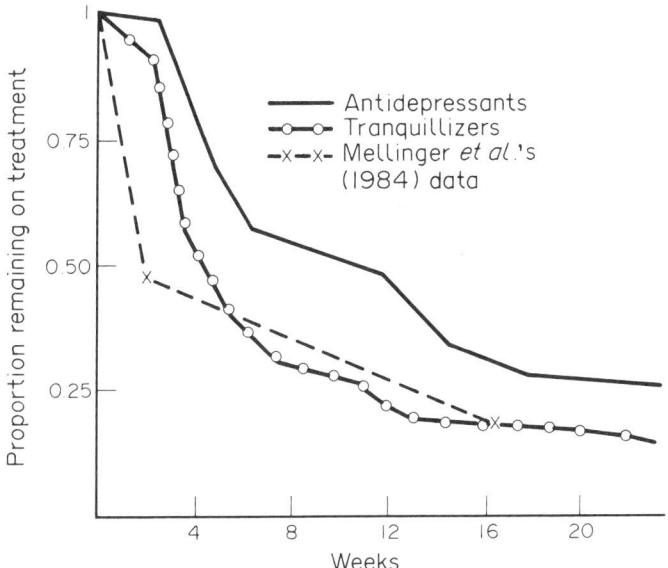

Figure 1. Survival distribution of duration of psychotropic drug use.

Fig. 1 shows the survival distributions according to the type of psychotropic drug prescribed at inception into the study. After six weeks, just over half of the patients on antidepressants were still receiving treatment, compared with about one-third of those on tranquillizers (virtually all of which were benzodiazepines). Just under 30% of the antidepressant recipients and just under 20% of the tranquillizer recipients were prescribed drugs for the entire six-month period. Also plotted on Fig. 1, for purposes of comparison, are the two points which can be derived from Mellinger et al.'s (32) data on self-reported 'longest period of daily use (i.e. consumption) during the past 12 months' of anti-anxiety agents. The disparities between the survival curves for the two-week point is striking, as is the similarity for the four-month point.

We then used survival analysis techniques to investigate factors which predicted continuation of treatment with psychotropic drugs (31). In so doing, we sought to extend the range of factors beyond those usually investigated: in addition to studying two characteristics of the *patients* (sex; age), we included two aspects of their *health status* (GPs' assessment of severity of symptoms at inception of treatment; presence or absence of physical illness), a measure of *social functioning* (GPs' assessment of social problems), three aspects of the *treatment* (type of psychotropic prescribed; past psychotropic drug use; whether or not drugs were requested by the patient), and the *passage of time*.

The effects of these factors on the survival distribution of drug use were first examined at a descriptive level, i.e. one at a time. At this level of analysis, severity of symptoms, type of psychotropic drug, and previous psychotropic drug use were each related to the duration of treatment (more severe, antidepressant prescription and a previous history of psychotropic use each indicating longer duration). There was also an association between increasing age and duration of treatment for tranquillizers but not for antidepressants, and an effect of sex (duration longer in women than men) only in those patients assessed by the GP as having significant social problems.

Such an analysis is sufficient for descriptive purposes (i.e. it allows us to answer such questions as 'do patients with characteristic X tend to receive treatment for longer

Table 2

Probability of discontinuing psychotropic drug treatment within the next two weeks (women only: estimated from the logistic model in Williams (31)

	Social problems identified by GP	Previous psychotropic drug use	
		No	Yes
At the beginning of treatment	None or one	0·34	0·21
	Two or more	0·45	0·11
After 4 months treatment	None or one	0·12	0·05
	Two or more	0·21	0·02

than those without it?), but is inadequate for explanatory purposes, since no account is taken of relationships between the predictor variables and possible interactive effects on the duration of drug use. Thus, we applied multiple logistic regression techniques, appropriate to the analysis of survival data.

Three significant effects were in the model of best fit. These were a history of *previous psychotropic drug use* (the presence of such a history decreased the likelihood of discontinuing treatment), an interactive effect of *sex and social problems* such that women in whom the GP identified social problems were less likely to discontinue treatment than either women without such problems or men), and the *passage of time* — the longer the duration of treatment, the less the chance of stopping.

These findings applied equally to patients on antidepressants and tranquillizers, and an example of the state of affairs predicted by the logistic model is given in Table 2. This shows the estimated probability of discontinuing psychotropic drug treatment within the next two weeks, at the beginning, and after four months of continuous treatment. A woman with social problems who has previously been treated with psychotropics has, compared with other women, little chance of early discontinuation of treatment at the start, and a negligible chance after four months of drug treatment.

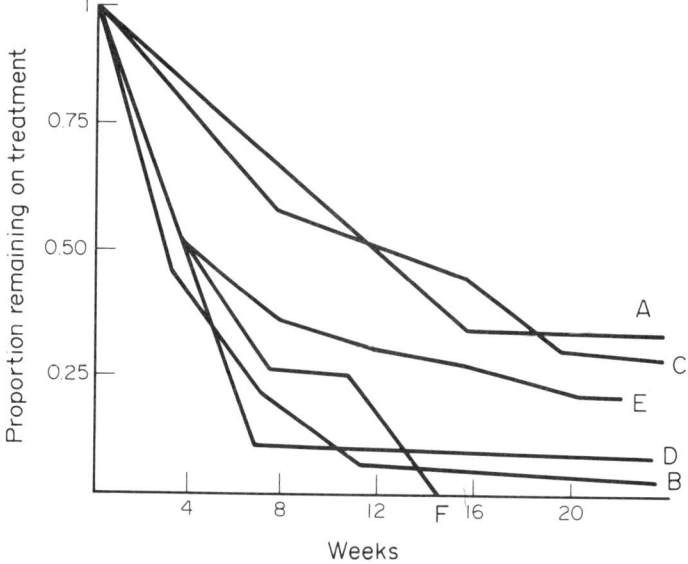

Figure 2. Survival distributions of duration of psychotropic drug use: between-doctor differences.

A further analysis was conducted to explore the differences between the doctors with regard to their patients' drug use. Fig. 2 demonstrates these differences: while all Dr F's patients stopped treatment within four months, about one-third of Dr A's patients were still receiving prescriptions after six months. Survivial analysis indicated that these differences were not due to differences between doctors with regard to the characteristics of their patients, nor to their patients' clinical pictures, nor to differences in aspects of the treatment (see Williams (31)). However, the effect of the passage of time on the probability of discontinuing treatment did vary between doctors, suggesting that some doctors may interact with their patients in such a way as to encourage, albeit not consciously, long-term use of benzodiazepines and other psychotropic drugs.

Findings such as these emphasize the need to consider factors other than the strictly demographic, clinical, or indeed pharmacological. They also provide support for the view of Cooperstock and Parnell (33) who, in a review of recent research on psychotropic drug use, identified a need for more studies from the point of view of the drug users themselves (both prescribers and recipients).

A cost-benefit approach to long-term benzodiazepine use

The need to consider the users' point of view is also apparent if a cost-benefit approach to long-term benzodiazepine use is adopted (34), since this strategy requires costs and benefits not only to be identified, but also to be quantified and valued (35).

Consider a general practitioner being consulted by a patient currently established on treatment with benzodiazepines. Unlike the decision to prescribe a drug which has definite and specific indications, the decision to continue treatment requires consideration of a wide variety of non-medical factors, and the patient may well be a more active participant in decision-making. Similar considerations may also apply to the prescription of other drugs whose indications are relatively broad, e.g. analgesics.

For the patient, potential benefits of continuing benzodiazepines may either be direct (e.g. improvements in well-being and/or social functioning) or may consist in the avoidance of disbenefit (e.g. the prevention of withdrawal phenomena in a pharmacologically-dependent patient). The second type is presumably more important in the context of long-term use. The benefits for the doctor of continuing to prescribe include the avoidance of alternative therapeutic effort (36) (patients also may seek to avoid potentially painful psychological exploration by demanding drug treatment), and the potential avoidance of conflict with a patient who wishes to continue drug treatment.

The costs for the doctor may well include anxiety engendered by the dissonance between the 'principles of good prescribing' and the problems encountered in practical prescribing in a social context. The potential costs to the patient of continued benzodiazepine use include not only immediate unwanted effects (such as cognitive impairment), but also temporally more distant consequences such as the possibility of an increased risk of accidents and drug-induced tissue damage (if indeed it occurs — see Tyrer (37)). In cost-benefit terms, these are regarded as '(dis)benefits in anticipation' (38), since although the drug is consumed now (and the benefit enjoyed now), the cost will be incurred, if at all, at some time in the future.

There is also another category of potential cost to the patient, in terms of self-esteem and self-image. Long-term users of tranquillizers are rarely neutral in their attitudes to their drugs (39,40), so that if patients perceive themselves to be 'dependent' or 'addicted', this may need to be considered in the cost-benefit equation.

As indicated above, the cost-benefit approach requires that costs and benefits, once identified, be quantified and valued (35). While the objective frequency and severity of the various potential costs and benefits of long-term benzodiazepine use is a matter for clinical research, it is clear that in decision-making, individuals act on their perception of information rather than on the information itself (41). The perceived or subjective probabilities (of occurrence of costs and benefits) thus assume greater importance: the extent to which these reflect the objective probabilities is a matter for empirical research.

The way in which patients and doctors value the costs and benefits is also important, and is likely to vary widely. For example, a doctor might be expected to value the avoidance of alternative therapeutic effort more highly than a patient will value the saving of medical time. Similarly, a patient who is indifferent to the notion of being dependent on tranquillizers may be expected to have a different value system from a psychiatrist such as Snaith (42) who opined that the prescribing of benzodiazepines should be forbidden by law. Furthermore, the possible long-term adverse consequences (the disbenefits in anticipation) will tend to be discounted and hence regarded as unimportant by patients (37), whereas they may be regarded as very important by doctors; however, this may well change over time, as suggested by some aspects of the growth of public concern about benzodiazepine use (12).

The views of long-term benzodiazepine users

The research on long-term use of benzodiazepines and other psychotropic drugs points to the importance of studying the point of view of the drug users themselves (doctors as well as their patients (43)) — a notion highlighted by considering the problem within a cost-benefit framework.

Doctors

Relatively few studies have focused on doctors. However, Gottlieb *et al.* (44) studied a group of psychiatrists, general physicians, and medical students with regard to their knowledge of, rather than attitudes about benzodiazepines and antidepressants. Using a multiple-choice questionnaire, they found that none of the respondents were 'sufficiently informed about, the diagnosis and psychotropic drug treatment of anxiety states and depressive syndromes'. In particular, the psychiatrists' scores on questions about the 'physiology, pharmacology and side effects of diazepam did not exceed those of medical house staff or medical students . . . their responses revealed a lack of familiarity with the properties of diazepam'.

Linn (45) used a postal questionnaire to assess the attitudes of both general practitioners and specialists in internal medicine to the use of benzodiazepines and other tranquillizers, and to relate these to the characteristics of the doctors themselves and of their practices. They were first asked to indicate their agreement to general statements about the use of tranquillizers, and the responses indicated considerable differences in opinion. Such heterogeneity was also apparent when the doctors were asked to assess the legitimacy of a number of situations in which a tranquillizer was used — 'opinion was well distributed through all categories of legitimacy'. Linn then studied the relationships between these attitudes and characteristics of the doctors and their practices, and two important relationships emerged. Firstly, doctors from a working-class background were more likely to be favourably disposed to the use of tranquillizers, and secondly, those doctors who were practising in relative isolation were also more likely to approve of the use of tranquillizers. The latter relationship is supported by Gabe and Williams' (46) finding that in urban areas, single-handed doctors exhibited the highest rates of tranquilizer prescribing.

Gabe and Lipshitz-Phillips (40) took a different approach — in-depth interviews with a small sample ($n = 14$) of general practitioners in London. Information was collected about the doctors' reasons for prescribing benzodiazepines and the factors which they felt influenced their decision to prescribe, as well as their views about patients' dependence on such drugs, and on alternatives to prescribing.

It was clear that in general, the doctors adopted a multifactorial view of benzodiazepine prescribing: while symptoms of anxiety and/or insomnia were universally mentioned, physical disorders (especially musculoskeletal) were also frequently cited as reasons for prescribing. Furthermore, most of the doctors mentioned patients' interpersonal and domestic problems as being important in influencing the decision while about one-third mentioned social structural factors such as work problems, poor housing, or financial difficulties. Most believed that they were more likely to prescribe benzodiazepines to working-class patients.

The doctors all said that they were aware of the dangers of patients becoming dependent on benzodiazepines, and seemed to be united in their concern to restrict their prescribing to the short-term management of crisis situations. The majority mentioned alternative strategies that they would propose to patients: these included counselling and support, the recommendation of relaxing social activities (such as yoga), and the possible involvement of other members of the primary care team.

Patients

It is only recently that investigators have begun to concern themselves in a systematic way with the views of the patients who use benzodiazepines or other tranquillizers on a long-term basis, and the impetus for such research has come primarily from social scientists rather than doctors. The methods used include postal surveys (28), structured interviews and questionnaires (17), in-depth semi-structured interviews (39,40,47,48), and group discussions (33). Two issues arising out of this research will be discussed here: long-term users' perceptions of the effects of the drugs; and their views as to their continued need for, as well as how they would cope without their drugs.

Do long-term users regard their drugs as helpful? It appears that in a general sense, most do (17,28). However, there is also evidence of considerable ambivalence: for example, 87% of respondents in Murray's (28) survey agreed with the statement 'I don't like taking these tablets but I could not manage without them'. Furthermore, when Gabe and Thorogood (48) asked women who were long-term users of benzodiazepines what they felt about taking the drugs, one-tenth of the sample emphasized the benefits and one-quarter the dangers, while the majority (about two-thirds) expressed mixed views. They also found that less ambivalence and fewer negative views were expressed by a sample of short-term users.

An important finding has been that when asked to specify the ways in which benzodiazepines and other tranquillizers are beneficial, long-term users frequently mention aspects of social functioning and performance. Table 3 shows the activities in which respondents expressed a need for drugs, as reported in Murray's (28) questionnaire survey of long-term psychotropic drug consumers and in Rodrigo

Table 3
Activities for which respondents felt a need for psychotropic drugs

	Current long-term users of psychotropic drugs (Murray (8)) $n = 183$	Current long-term users of benzodiazepines (Rodrigo et al. (17)) $n = 64$
	No %	No %
Travelling	81 (44)	7 (11)
Shopping	78 (43)	4 (6)
Mixing with people	75 (41)	7 (11)
Running the home	65 (36)	8 (13)
Work	61 (33)	16 (25)
Family problems	6 1(33)	1 (2)
Marriage	40 (22)	3 (5)
Money matters	20 (11)	2 (3)
Housing problems	13 (7)	1 (2)

et al.'s (17) interview study of long-term benzodiazepine consumers in a south London general practice. There are clearly marked differences between the two studies (which may well be accounted for by the nature of the samples and the methods used), but together, they testify to the extent to which users regard benzodiazepines and other psychotropic drugs as having a social as well as a purely clinical function. A similar finding emerged from Cooperstock and Lennard's (33) series of group discussions with long-term benzodiazepine users, while over half of the long-term psychotropic drug users interviewed by Helman (39) felt that withdrawal of the drugs would have a bad effect on their social relationships.

Of the current long-term users surveyed by Murray (28) 58 per cent said they would find it 'very difficult' to manage without their drugs, and a further 33% claimed that they would not be able to manage at all. A similar picture emerges from Rodrigo et al.'s (17) study: while a smaller proportion (17%) said they could not 'do without', more than half (54%) of the long-term benzodiazepine consumers believed that they would need to take their drugs either for 'years' or indefinitely.

An important aspect of the long-term use of prescribed drugs is the patient's perceptions of their doctors' attitude. Murray (28) found a 'widespread belief in the general practitioner's acquiescence in continued drug taking'—81% of her respondents claimed that their doctors either wished them to continue or did not mind. Similarly, in Rodrigo et al.'s study, 33 patients (52%) had no idea as to the doctor's views, and a further 24 (38%) believed that he encouraged their use; 52 of the patients claimed that their GP had never suggested that they stop the drug.

In both studies, users were asked to suggest alternative strategies that they would use if the drugs were not available. In both, the predominant strategy was the consumption of some alternative substance—other drugs, alcohol, and herbal remedies being the most frequently mentioned. Similarly, cigarette smoking was regarded as an alternative resource by the women interviewed by Gabe and Thorogood (48). In Rodrigo et al.'s study, 11 patients (17%) could envisage no possible alternative to benzodiazepines, and some expressed a fear of becoming mentally ill without their tablets.

In the latter study, an attempt was also made to assess patients' valuation of benzodiazepines: they were first asked to nominate their five favourite leisure activities, and then to indicate how many, and which, of these they would be willing to forego in order to ensure a continued supply of drugs. Twenty-nine of the patients (45%) considered the drug more important than all the activities they nominated in that they claimed to be willing to give them all up in order to remain on the drug.

Some of these findings on users' perceptions and views can be integrated by using the concept of *meaning* — i.e. 'the interpretation a person gives to an object or event in his or her life' (49). This approach was used by Helman (39) and also by Gabe (40, 48), who has developed the concepts 'lifeline' and 'standby' to describe the meaning of benzodiazepines to consumers. Those who viewed their drugs as a lifeline felt them to be 'something which they needed to take regularly and depended on' simply to keep going in the face of chronic, unresolved problems. Others viewed their drugs as a standby, to be kept in reserve and used occasionally to meet some short-lived crisis, while a minority of their respondents characterized their drug-taking behaviour in terms of both these meanings.

Helman (39) conducted in-depth interviews wtih 50 long-term (6 months or more) benzodiazepine users. He found, on the basis of their beliefs, attitudes and expectations concerning the drugs, that 'long-term users of psychotropics can be classified into three main groups — "tonic", "food" and "fuel".'

Patients classified as 'tonic' (about one-third of the sample) were those who expressed maximum control over the drug, its dosage, and when it was to be used, tending to use the drugs on a prn rather than a regular basis. They placed the site of action of the drug on themselves rather than on their relationships, and tended to have more anti-drug views than the other groups. Patients classified as 'fuel' (some two-fifths of those interviewed) expressed a variable degree of control over their medication, but nonetheless felt that the drug played an important and constant part in their daily lives. Its maximum effect was thought to be on their relationships with others: in some cases, the drug was seen as an essential constituent of the patients' relationships. Helman used the concept of 'fuel', in the sense that without the drug, 'the patient would not disintegrate but would just not function in conformity with familial and social expectations'.

The third group of patients (about one-fifth of the sample), for whom benzodiazepines were conceptualized as a 'food', expressed least control over the drug, its ingestion, and over life generally. Helman noted that their psychological dependence was as much on the medical profession as on the drug. Furthermore, the drugs were seen by this group as acting both on the patient's emotional state and on social relationships: without it, both would disintegrate. Helman applied the concept of 'food' to these patients' drug use, since without it, they would not survive as an independent, sane person.

Conclusion

Long-term use of benzodiazepines and other psychotropic drugs remains a major feature of general practice. It is clear that the phenomenon should not be conceptualized only within a pharmacological or a strictly clinical context. Indeed, the work described above testifies to the importance of taking the users' own views into account, and suggests that this would be a fruitful field for further exploration with regard to understanding and managing long-term psychotropic drug use.

Acknowledgments

The author is supported by the Department of Health and Social Security. Work undertaken by him and his colleagues forms part of a DHSS-funded programme of research conducted by the General Practice Research Unit, under the direction of Professor Michael Shepherd. Grateful thanks are due to Mr Jon Gabe for his comments on an earlier version of this paper.

References

(1) Parish PA. The prescribing of psychotropic drugs in general practice. *J Roy Coll Gen Pract* 1971; **21** (Suppl 4): 1-77.
(2) Trethowan WH. Pills for personal problems. *Br Med J* 1985; **iii**: 749-51.
(3) Williams P. Recent trends in the prescribing of psychotropic drugs. *Health Trends* 1980; **17**: 845-51.
(4) Williams P. Patterns of psychotropic drug use. *Soc Sci Med* 1983a; **17**: 845-51.
(5) Skegg DCG, Doll R, Perry J. Use of medicines in general practice. *Br Med J* 1977; **i**: 1561-3.
(6) Dunnell K, Cartwright A. *Medicine takers, prescribers and hoarders*. London: Routledge and Kegan Paul, 1972.
(7) Murray J, Dunn G, Williams P, Tarnopolsky A. Factors affecting the consumption of psychotropic drugs. *Psychol Med* 1981; **11**: 551-60.
(8) Anderson R. Prescribed medicines—who takes what? *J Epidemiol Comm Hlth* 1980; **34**: 299-304.
(9) Marks J. The benzodiazepines—for good or for evil? *Neuropsychobiology* 1983; **10**: 115-26.
(10) Marks J. The benzodiazepines: an international perspective. *J Psychoactive Drugs* 1983; **15**: 137-49.
(11) Williams P, Bellantuono C, Fiorio R, Tansella M. Psychotropic drug use in Italy: national trends and regional differences. *Psychol Med*; 1986; **16**: 841-50.
(12) Gabe J, Williams P. Tranquillizer use: a historical perspective. In: Gabe J, Williams P, eds. *Tranquillisers: social, psychological and clinical perspectives*. London: Tavistock Publications, 1986: 3-17.
(13) Woodcock J. Long-term consumers of psychotropic drugs. In: Balint M, Marinker M, Woodcock J, eds. *Treatment or diagnosis*. London: Tavistock Publications, 1970: 147-76.
(14) Cooperstock R. Psychotropic drug use among women. *Can Med Assoc J* 1976; **115**: 760-3.
(15) Cooperstock R. Sex differences in psychotropic drug use. *Soc Sci Med* 1978; **12B**: 179-86.
(16) Mellinger GD, Balter MB, Uhlenhuth EH. Prevalence and correlates of long-term regular use of anxiolytics. *JAMA* 1984; **251**: 375-9.
(17) Rodrigo EK, King M, Williams P. Long-term tranquillizer use in a south London general practice. Research report, Institute of Psychiatry, 1987.
(18) Mellinger GD, Balter MB, Uhlenhuth EH, Cisin IH, Manheimer DI, Rickels K. Evaluating a household survey measure of psychic distress. *Psychol Med* 1983; **13**: 607-21.
(19) Goldberg D, Cooper B, Eastwood MR, Kedward HB, Shepherd M. A standardised psychiatric interview for use in community surveys. *J Prev Soc Med* 1970; **24**: 18-23.
(20) Marks J, Goldberg D, Hillier VE. Determinants of the ability of general practitioners to detect psychiatric disorder. *Psychol Med* 1979; **9**: 337-53.
(21) Skuse DH, Williams P. Screening for psychiatric disorder in general practice. *Psychol Med* 1984; **14**: 365-77.
(22) Weissman MM, Klerman GL. The chronic depressive in the community: unrecognised and poorly treated. *Comprehen Psych* 1977; **18**: 523-32.

(23) Gullick EL, King LJ. Appropriateness of drugs prescribed by primary care physicians for depressed outpatients. *J Affect Disorders* 1979; **1**: 55-8.
(24) Weissman MM, Myers JK, Thompson WD. Depression and its treatment in a US urban community. *Arch Gen Psych* 1981; **38**: 417-21.
(25) Solow C. Psychotropic drugs in somatic disorder. *Int J Psych Med* 1975; **6**: 267-82.
(26) Williams P. Physical ill-health and psychotropic drug prescription: a review. *Psychol Med* 1978; **8**: 683-93.
(27) Murray J, Williams P, Clare AW. Health and social characteristics of long-term psychotropic drug takers. *Soc Sci Med* 1982; **16**: 1595-8.
(28) Murray J. Long-term psychotropic drug taking and the process of withdrawal. *Psychol Med* 1981; **11**: 853-8.
(29) Belloc NB, Breslow L, Hochstim JR. Measurement of physical health in a general population survey. *Am J Epidemiol* 1971; **93**: 328-36.
(30) Williams P, Murray J, Clare AW. A longitudinal study of psychotropic drug prescription. *Psychol Med* 1982; **12**: 201-6.
(31) Williams P. Factors influencing the duration of treatment with psychotropic drugs in general practice: a survival analysis approach. *Psychol Med* 1983; **13**: 623-33.
(32) Mellinger GD, Balter MB, Uhlenhuth EH. Anti-anxiety agents: duration of use and characteristics of users in the USA. *Curr Med Res Opinion* 1984; **8** (Suppl 4): 21-36.
(33) Cooperstock R, Lennard H. Some social meanings of tranquillizer use. *Sociol Health Illness* 1979; **1**: 331-47.
(34) Williams P, Rodrigo EK. An economic approach to benzodiazepine use. Unpublished paper, Institute of Psychiatry, 1987.
(35) Drummond M. *Principles of economic appraisal in health care*. Oxford: Oxford University Press, 1980.
(36) Marinker M. The doctor's role in prescribing. *J Roy Coll Gen Pract* 1973; **23** (Suppl 2): 26-9.
(37) Tyrer P. Benzodiazepines on trial. *Br Med J* 1984; **288**: 1101-2.
(38) Cohen D. Utility model of preventive behaviour. *J Epidemiol Comm Health* 1984; **38**: 61-5.
(39) Helman C. Tonic, fuel and food: social and symbolic aspects of the long-term use of psychotropic drugs. *Soc Sci Med* 1981; **15B**: 521-33.
(40) Gabe J, Lipshitz-Phillips S. Evil necessity? The meaning of benzodiazepine use for women patients from one general practice. *Sociol Health Illness* 1982; **4**: 201-9.
(41) Shelly MW, Bryan GL. *Human judgement and optimality*. New York: Wiley, 1964.
(42) Snaith RP. Benzodiazepines on trial. *Br Med J* 1984; **288**: 1379.
(43) Cooperstock R, Parnell P. Research on psychotropic drug use: a review of findings and methods. *Soc Sci Med* 1982; **16**: 1179-96.
(44) Gottlieb RM, Nappi T, Strain JJ. The physician's knowledge of psychotropic drugs. *Am J Psych* 1978; **135**: 29-32.
(45) Linn LS. Physician characteristics and attitudes toward legitimate use of psychotherapeutic drugs. *J Health Soc Behav* 1971; **12**: 132-40.
(46) Gabe J, Williams P. Rural tranquility? Urban-rural differences in tranquilliser prescription. *Soc Sci Med* 1986; **22**: 1059-66.
(47) Gabe J, Lipshitz-Phillips S. Tranquillisers as social control? *Sociol Rev* 1984; **32**: 524-6.
(48) Gabe J, Thorogood N. Tranquillisers as a resource. In: Gabe J, Williams P, eds. *Tranquillisers: social, psychological and clinical perspectives*. London: Tavistock Publications, 1986: 244-69.
(49) Gabe J, Williams P. The meaning of tranquilliser use: introduction. In: Gabe J, Williams P, eds. *Tranquillisers: social, psychological and clinical perspectives*. London: Tavistock Publications, 1986: 197-8.

Discussion

Dr Beary asked about the average age when people took their first benzodiazepine, because the implication was that a drug started in, say, the late 30s would accumulate over the years. Although it was older women who were taking such medication, it was in younger women that there was an increase in alcoholism, and these might be the most important group.

Dr Williams replied that only a small proportion of benzodiazepine users continued to long-term use, and they were predominantly older people.

Professor Lader said he had seen data which suggested that whereas in the late 1960s or early 1970s, one in three prescriptions for benzodiazepines were long-term, the figure was now about two-thirds or three-quarters, but the reliability of those data was uncertain. He had been surprised to find in Dr Williams' study, that none of the 24 chronic users had the label of anxiety state, and believed that many problems could be circumvented or minimized if patients with depression were not given benzodiazepines. He wondered whether there was a group of neurotic depressives, put on benzodiazepines, who were at a particular risk of continuing, or whether the diagnosis changed over time, starting as an anxiety state and then developing into depression as a result of treatment.

Professor Clare pointed out that these were the diagnostic categories used by psychiatrists; general practitioners tended to use a different terminology.

Dr Williams agreed that these were categories imposed by psychiatrists. As to the reasons for the initial prescription, seven of the patients said it was for depression, 11 for anxiety and other reasons were insomnia, muscle tension, and pain; of these, insomnia was the largest category.

Dr Marks said that in his experience in Liverpool, 'depression' was a term commonly used because patients had learned that it was an acceptable label: if they complained about their real problem—marital or financial for instance—no-one paid attention. When general practitioners referred patients to the local psychiatric department, the prescriptions might be continued, or changed, or increased. However, there was a marked difference between two local psychiatric hospitals: one tended to increase benzodiazepine prescriptions, and the other regularly put patients on behavioural withdrawal regimes. This influence would be interesting to study.

Professor Rickels returned to the problem of diagnosis. Of 119 patients interviewed in his clinic who were long-term benzodiazepine users (average duration eight years), only a third had a generalized anxiety diagnosis, including some with dysthymic disorder and some with anxiety; about a third had major depressive disorder, 25% panic disorder, and 10% no psychiatric diagnosis. Deciding on appropriate treatment and discontinuing inappropriate treatment where necessary is an important step in preventing addiction to benzodiazepines.

Dr Tyrer was concerned that after four months antidepressants were prescribed much more commonly than benzodiazepines. Volunteer groups such as Tranx Release tended to make little distinction between antidepressants and benzodiazepines, and indeed many of their consumers regarded them as the same. Although he recommended antidepressants more frequently than benzodiazepines for this population, he was worried that large numbers of long-term consumers of antidepressants would result, in the same way as had happened with benzodiazepines.

Professor Lader said that benzodiazepines were actually more effective than antidepressants in that kind of patient. He had recently reviewed a number of trials comparing cognitive therapy with pharmacotherapy, and it was clear that simple measures were often effective; many patients did not need drugs at all. There was also evidence that about two-thirds of the prescriptions for anxiolytics were unnecessary.

Mr Taylor referred to the numbers of prescriptions, and suspected that people were generally taking the tablets very intermittently; though many prescriptions were repeats, the idea of continuous consumption was often incorrect. The cost of a prescription was marginal, compared with perhaps £20 or £30 an hour for cognitive therapy.

Professor Freeman asked how cognitive therapy could be provided for very large numbers of people; he found difficulty in obtaining it for one person.

Professor Lader thought that general practitioners could be trained, or a system set up which reimbursed them for psychological services. If general practitioners could provide obstetric services, for which they were paid separately, they could be paid to provide psychological services, or at least to supervise such services. He was not suggesting that they should necessarily carry out the treatment themselves.

Dr Marks said that his practice used the community psychiatric nurses (CPNs) who worked very effectively with groups of patients, using cognitive techniques. The Department of Psychiatry had put community psychiatric nurses at the service of four general practice health centres, each with six doctors. During surgery, any appropriate cases were sent through to the CPN, and were dealt with in groups, either in the centre or in the Department of Psychiatry, with two sessions each week. There was now a standard four-week course, which was proving very efficient, approaching a 90% success rate.

Dr Wheatley felt that it was not a question of training general practitioners or even of rewarding them for time-consuming work; it was the time itself that was the problem. The general practitioner had not got the time to spend perhaps 20 or 30 min with each patient.

Professor Clare referred back to the earlier comment that anxiolytics were not specific. It was clear that while psychiatrists had a tendency to think that benzodiazepines should be used, if at all, for anxiety neurosis, phobic states, or panic disorders, in practice they were used for a variety of complaints, while the patients thought they were used to help them cope with social difficulties.

Psychiatric indications for benzodiazepines

KARL RICKELS and EDWARD SCHWEIZER

Department of Psychiatry, University of Pennsylvania, Philadelphia, Pennsylvania 19104, USA

Since their introduction over 25 years ago, benzodiazepines have been among the most widely prescribed compounds in medicine. This can be attributed both to their enormous spectrum of effectiveness (as anxiolytics, sedatives, muscle relaxants, anticonvulsants) and to their relative safety. In psychiatry they rapidly took the place of barbiturates and meprobamate as the agents of choice for the treatment of insomnia and of all varieties of anxiety. That very effectiveness and safety created, perhaps, a too uncritical climate of clinical acceptance, and a tendency to prescribe benzodiazepines almost as a therapeutic reflex. This 'honeymoon' period lasted well over a decade, and only came to an end in the late 1970s, with a growing awareness of the potential for physical dependence and risk of withdrawal with chronic use. This awareness, coupled with surveys that revealed the extent to which a sector of the public had come to rely on benzodiazepines, served significantly to alter public attitudes towards the use of tranquillizers (1).

The hue and cry in the past decade over the possible liability of patients to develop dependence has probably been overstated, but it has forced a reconsideration of what are proper indications for the use of benzodiazepines in psychiatry. The current paper will be restricted to consideration of their use in insomnia and formal anxiety disorders.

It is a truism in medicine that indications for treatment should be dictated by diagnosis, but when it comes to management of anxiety, this has often been honoured only in the breach. Yet diagnosis is especially important when it comes to treating anxiety, which can exist either as a primary diagnosis—an autonomous syndrome with its own heritable vulnerability, natural history, etc—or as a secondary set of symptoms complicating another primary clinical diagnosis (whether medical or psychiatric). An illustration from an ongoing study (2) on chronic benzodiazepine use highlights the possible consequences of not first establishing diagnosis in a symptomatically anxious patient. A substantial percentage of the patients chronically dependent on benzodiazepines whom we have evaluated had been prescribed this medication without ever having received a careful initial diagnosis, and often, there was no apparent attempt even to make one. More attention to initial diagnosis might have resulted in more judicious use of benzodiazepines, or in use of alternative medication, with consequently less risk of long-term dependence.

The benzodiazepines in current clinical practice, edited by Hugh Freeman and Yvonne Rue, 1987: Royal Society of Medicine Services International Congress and Symposium Series No. 114, published by Royal Society of Medicine Services Limited.

Table 1

Major indications for benzodiazepine use (DSM-III) diagnoses

Generalized anxiety disorder
Atypical anxiety disorder
Panic disorder
Post-traumatic stress disorder
Adjustment disorders with anxious mood
Somatization disorder
Disorders of initiating or maintaining sleep (DIMS)–insomnia

Benzodiazepines certainly have a role to play in management of the symptomatic anxiety of medical disorders, and they have also been used in the adjunctive treatment of other psychiatric conditions, such as the psychoses. But these are less well established uses.

Table 1 lists the anxiety and sleep disorders for which benzodiazepines are most frequently prescribed. Once a diagnosis has been made, how does a clinician arrive at the decision to prescribe? Choice of treatment must be guided by the need to alleviate a patient's distressing symptoms and to improve his/her functioning. Both clinical experience and controlled research clearly support the efficacy of benzodiazepines in affording relief of anxiety and in achieving the other therapeutic goals (3). Fig. 1 summarizes the response to diazepam versus placebo in a four-week double-blind trial in anxious patients seen in two different settings: family practice and private psychiatric practice (4). In both settings, benzodiazepines offered a significant advantage over placebo, but it is of note that placebo itself was associated with significant relief of anxiety symptoms.

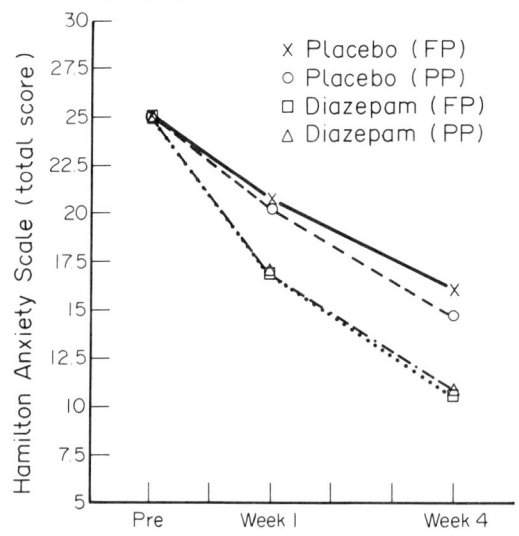

Figure 1. Diazepam and placebo in family practice and private psychiatric practice in patients with anxiety.

This latter observation underscores the importance in treating anxiety of considering non-specific curative factors such as patient expectancy, supportive contact with a doctor, and that often neglected healer—the passage of time. Catalan et al. (5) have provided strong prospective evidence for the value of such factors: 91 patients seen in general practice and recommended for benzodiazepine treatment were randomized to receive either a benzodiazepine or very brief counselling from their doctor. Seven-month follow-up revealed significant and parallel improvement in the anxiety symptoms in both groups, without increased demands being made on the time of doctors by the non-benzodiazepine group. One may conclude that for patients presenting with low-to-moderate levels of anxiety, social and psychological therapies are appropriate, and even desirable alternatives to drug therapy. In fact, little is lost and much is often gained by not rushing headlong into drug treatment merely to palliate the patient. An extra week or so of observation, a supportive and empathic attitude, and an attempt to understand the nature of a patient's underlying problems and life stresses will often yield much relief.

On the other hand, such a cautious approach can be carried too far and become a dogmatic reluctance to prescribe any benzodiazepine. This backlash is as ill-founded as the reflexive use of benzodiazepines, or their prescription as a panacea. The safety and efficacy of benzodiazepines in anxiety states should argue for a highly favourable cost/benefit/risk ratio, when compared to many psychotherapeutic approaches to anxiety. Very often, judicious use of a benzodiazepine constitutes the treatment of choice, and not merely a treatment of last resort.

When benzodiazepines are being considered as a treatment option, it is useful to remember some of the predictors of favourable response to treatment that have been gleaned from studies over the years. How well a patient responds to a benzodiazepine varies greatly in light of these factors: short duration of illness, presence of an identifiable stressor, high levels of somatic and psychic anxiety, and low levels of depressive, phobic, and hypochondriacal complaints all predict favourable anxiolytic response (6,7). Chronicity of symptoms and neuroticism as an enduring personality trait both make for a less favourable response, but even 50% of chronically anxious patients will not only achieve a remission in anxiety symptoms by six weeks, but will stay symptom-free when blindly switched to eight weeks of placebo (8).

While most benzodiazepines are considered not very effective in the treatment of major depressive disorders, clinical research suggests that alprazolam may possibly be an exception, at least in the treatment of outpatients (9,10). Similarly, the presence of crescendo anxiety attacks has also been considered to suggest a diagnosis (panic disorder) with reduced responsiveness to benzodiazepines—again with the notable exception of alprazolam (11). Recently, though, other high-potency benzodiazepines such as clonazepam and lorazepam, and even low potency benzodiazepines such as diazepam have demonstrated anti-panic effects, especially if prescribed in higher doses than is standard for non-panic anxiety (12). The question whether use of benzodiazepines will prove less effective in panic states complicated by agoraphobia awaits the results of further research.

The treatment of panic disorder, with or without agoraphobia, may frequently necessitate treatment for several months or longer, but even in these circumstances, short-term treatment should be attempted first. If indeed a patient is in need of prolonged benzodiazepine therapy for panic disorder, other treatment options such as imipramine or a monoamine oxidase inhibitor should be reviewed. Assessment of potential benefit from long-term benzodiazepines must be weighed against the increased risk of withdrawal on discontinuation; a very gradual and well-managed tapering of the drug will serve to minimize discomfort in the vast majority of patients.

Generalized anxiety disorder and panic are the classic psychiatric indications for benzodiazepine treatment, but when are benzodiazepines indicated for that vast array of more transient and situational anxiety states? An understanding of the role of benzodiazepines in the optimal management of insomnia may shed some light on how optimally to manage the common varieties of anxiety.

Table 2
NIMH consensus conference: drugs and insomnia

Type of insomnia	Treatment	Duration of treatment
Transient insomnia (situational stress, e.g. jet lag)	No treatment or hypnotics	1–3 days
Short-term insomnia (situational stress e.g. acute personal loss, often related to work, family life or serious medical illness)	Hypnotics + sleep hygiene and non-drug procedures	Up to 3 weeks
Long-term insomnia (many causes; needs extensive medical evaluation)	1. Initial approach — non-drug and treatment of underlying medical or psychiatric illness; 2. Trial of hypnotics.	<1 month; if longer — intermediate rather than continuous

The 1983 NIMH Consensus Conference on Drugs and Insomnia (13) descriptively sub-divided insomnias into three main categories (Table 2). The treatment recommendations were different for each category.

Transient insomnia was delineated as a condition found in normal sleepers who were experiencing an acute situational stress, usually lasting not more than one to three days (e.g. admission to hospital for operation, jet lag, etc.). Where elected, treatment with hypnotics should be performed with the smallest dose possible, and a rapidly eliminated hypnotic be preferred.

Short-term insomnia was also defined as being related to situational stress, but the disruption of sleep was more persistent. Therefore, a brief trial of an hypnotic was felt to be beneficial, as long as this trial was clearly a part of an overall treatment approach that emphasized improvement of sleep hygiene, along with other non-drug procedures. Any drug treatment should be time-limited, not lasting longer than a few weeks.

Long-term or chronic insomnia was felt to necessitate an intensive differential diagnostic work-up. Psychiatric conditions, drug and alcohol abuse, chronic medical illness, and sleep disorders such as nocturnal myoclonus, sleep apnoea or delayed sleep phase syndrome have to be considered before a patient can be successfully treated. Some disagreement was reported about the management of chronic insomnia. In general, it was proposed to use non-drug strategies first and to treat the primary illness, if one is found to be present. Non-drug strategies might include exercise, decreased intake of caffeine, elimination of alcohol and recreational drugs, training in relaxation exercises, development of sleep rituals, elimination of daytime napping, and careful review of a patient's general sleep hygiene. Only if these approaches are not successful is the judicious use of hypnotics recommended, and then for no longer than one month at a time.

A parallel can be drawn between long-term insomnia and generalized anxiety and panic: both are autonomous and self-perpetuating clinical states that go beyond any precipitating stressor, and both require aggressive treatment strategies. These are usually ones in which benzodiazepines have a role to play, but only after a careful differential diagnosis has been undertaken. On the other hand, short-term anxiety states are like the short-term and transient insomnias, in that they are much less autonomous and, by definition, more situationally linked to an identifiable stressor. As a result, the focus must be on the patient's life circumstances, external stressors, and the individual's standard means of coping. Attention to coping strategies is very important, since such habits can be regarded as the equivalent for anxiety of sleep hygiene for insomnia.

Next to establishing a diagnosis, the proper application of benzodiazepines in psychiatry hinges on how well the drug can be employed as a useful additional tool, to facilitate a more rapid return to a patient's own successful coping. However, to view them as a cure-all, instead of as a tool of enormous yet limited potential, is to create a tyranny of psychological dependence, which may be even harder to break than any physical dependence which may subsequently develop.

An interesting confirmation of this comes from the research of Catalan et al. (5), who found that the one group of patients who did poorly when randomized to non-drug treatment of their anxiety consisted of those who had developed a longstanding habit of self-medication with over-the-counter drugs—alcohol and cigarettes. These had become their prime means of coping, whereas benzodiazepines should be used in a way that facilitates a return to normal coping, not substitutes for it.

It might therefore be helpful to summarize some principles we have found useful in prescribing benzodiazepines for psychiatric indications (Table 3). Points 1 and 2 have already been elaborated on. Point 3 emphasizes that the prescribing doctor should have a clear sense of what target symptoms he is treating, should track the improvement of those symptoms over time, and should have a time-frame in mind for an adequate treatment period. Too often, clinicians have used benzodiazepines in a dismissive way to silence the 'background noise' of somatic or insomniac complaints in a treatment relationship. A recent survey (12) suggests that the somatically anxious patient may indeed resort to consultation with a doctor at a rate that is many times greater than his non-anxious counterpart. This argues for a collaborative effort on the part of both doctor and patient to understand properly the anxious basis of the patient's symptoms and to use benzodiazepines, where appropriate, to treat the anxiety aggressively.

Point 4 is a reminder that benzodiazepines should be titrated to the lowest possible dose that provides maximal relief of anxiety with the least adverse effects. The side-effects of benzodiazepines have been discussed at length elsewhere (15). Tolerance develops within a week or two to psychomotor and sedative effects, but until then, dosing after meals, dividing the dose, or other clinical manoeuvres usually suffice to make such side-effects tolerable for most patients. However, tolerance does not develop to the amnesic effects of benzodiazepines (16).

Given virtually identical profiles of pharmacological activity, the choice of benzodiazepines depends largely on pharmacokinetic considerations; the main

Table 3

Principles of benzodiazepine use in anxiety

1. Establish a diagnosis.
2. Treatment is collaborative with benzodiazepines being presented in terms of:
    a) relative benefits and risks
    b) one of several treatment options
3. Establish clear treatment goals in terms of both target symptoms and a time-frame for duration of benzodiazepine therapy.
4. Titrate benzodiazepines to the minimum effective dose.
5. Review achievement of treatment goals in first 2 weeks: lack of clear improvement should cause one to reconsider both the diagnosis and the treatment chosen.
6. If long-term benzodiazepine treatment is agreed upon, continued use should be regularly reassessed, and discontinuation of the benzodiazepines should be by gradual tapering.

exception is the weight of existing evidence favouring alprazolam in the treatment of panic disorder. Speed of absorption and rapidity of distribution, which in turn is a function of lipophilicity, is of more concern when benzodiazepines are being used acutely, or in an as-needed fashion. Elimination half-life becomes of greater concern with more chronic use, when active metabolites contribute considerably to persistent clinical effect (3).

Point 5 recalls research (7) which demonstrates that response to benzodiazepines usually occurs within the first two weeks of treatment. In fact, of patients who were unimproved after one week of benzodiazepine treatment, only 20% eventually showed any response, so that response after one week is one of the best predictors of ultimate treatment outcome. Lack of response should prompt a critical reconsideration of the diagnosis, especially bearing in mind the possibility of having missed an atypically presenting affective illness, or an Axis II personality disorder (DSM III). Alternatively, examination of the psychosocial context of a patient's anxious symptoms may reveal circumstances that require proportionately more psychological intervention, and a proportionately smaller role for a benzodiazepine. Treatment resistance in anxiety is only occasionally due to inadequate blood levels in the face of adequate dosing, so that although assessment of the plasma level of benzodiazepine occasionally pays off, by uncovering a rapid metabolizer, more often than not treatment resistance is an indication for a thorough diagnostic reassessment.

Point 6 indicates the need for caution about the risks of long-term benzodiazepine treatment. Surveys (e.g. 17) show that 1·6% of American adults have used a benzodiazepine for a year or longer. In the light of research (2,8) suggesting that physical dependence and withdrawal reactions on discontinuation can occur even at low-to-moderate doses, a fairly large number of patients are potentially at risk. However, this is manageable as long as discontinuation of the benzodiazepine is conducted very slowly, and with an awareness of what to expect.

Whether long-term benzodiazepine treatment is indicated in the first place obviously depends on the individual clinical situation. Partial or inadequate treatment response should prompt a reconsideration of diagnosis, and a possible switch to treatment with alternative medication such as an antidepressant. In such a clinical situation, continued use of benzodiazepine *faute de mieux* is probably unwise. If a serious or recurrent anxiety condition such as panic disorder or a chronic anxiety state is present and seems to require long-term treatment, it should only be instituted: (1) after fully apprising the patient of benefits, risks and treatment options; (2) in the context of efforts to equip the patient with a greater behavioural control over his symptoms; and (3) at the lowest effective daily dose, with the understanding that periodic review of the need for the medication, and attempts to taper it, should be made.

Over the years, benzodiazepines have proved to be enormously safe and effective medications. Their much publicized faults are less in the drug than in ourselves — how we as clinicians have used them. Careful attention to diagnostic indications for their use, and a clear recognition that benzodiazepines constitute a tool and not a panacea will go a long way towards maximizing their effectiveness and minimizing adverse effects.

References

(1) Clinthorne JK, Cisin IH, Balter MB, Mellinger GD, Uhlenhuth EH. Changes in popular attitudes and beliefs about tranquillizers. *Arch Gen Psych* 1986; **43**: 527–32.

(2) Rickels K, Case WG, Schweizer EE, Swenson C, Fridman RB. Low-dose dependence in chronic benzodiazepine users: A preliminary report on 119 patients. *Psychopharmacol Bull* 1986; **22** (no. 2); 407-15.
(3) Greenblatt DJ, Shader RI, Abernethy DR: Medical Intelligence. Drug Therapy. Current status of benzodiazepines (Parts I and II). *N Engl J Med* 1983; **309**: 354-8 and 410-16.
(4) Rickels K. To the Editor. Treatment of benzodiazepine dependence. *Med J Aust* 1987; **146**: 112.
(5) Catalan J, Gath D, Edmonds G, Ennis J, Bond A, Martin P. The effects of non-prescribing of anxiolytics in general practice. *Br J Psych* 1984; **144**: 593-610.
(6) Rickels K. Use of antianxiety agents in anxious outpatients. *Psychopharmacology* 1978; **58**: 1-17.
(7) Downing RW, Rickels K. Early treatment response in anxious outpatients treated with diazepam. *Acta Psych Scand* 1985; **72**: 522-8.
(8) Rickels K, Case WG, Downing RW, Winokur A. Long-term diazepam therapy and clinical outcome. *JAMA* 1983; **250**: 767-71.
(9) Feighner JP, Aden GC, Fabre LF, Rickels K, Smith WT. Comparison of alprazolam, imipramine, and placebo in the treatment of depression. *JAMA* 1983; **249**: 3057-64.
(10) Rickels K, Feighner JP, Smith WT. Alprazolam, amitriptyline, doxepin, and placebo in the treatment of depression. *Arch Gen Psychiatry* 1985; **42**: 134-41.
(11) Rickels K, Schweizer EE: Current pharmacotherapy of anxiety and panic. In: Meltzer H, Bunney B, Coyle J *et al.* eds. *Psychopharmacology. 3rd generation of progress*. New York: Raven Press, in press.
(12) Dunner DL, Ishiki D, Avery DH, Wilson LG, Hyde TF. Effect of alprazolam and diazepam on anxiety and panic attacks in panic disorder: A controlled study. *J Clin Psych* 1986; **47**: 458-60.
(13) Consensus Conference: drugs and insomnia. The use of medication to promote sleep. *JAMA* 1984; **251**: 2410-14.
(14) Smith GR, Monson RA, Ray DC. Patients with multiple unexplained symptoms. Their characteristics, functional health, and health care utilization. *Arch Intern Med* 1986; **146**: 69-72.
(15) Rickels K, Schweizer E, Lucki I: Benzodiazepine side effects. In: Hales RE, Frances AJ, eds. *Psychiatry update, vol. 6. American Psychiatric Association Annual Review*. Washington: American Psychiatric Association Press, 1987: 781-801.
(16) Lucki I, Rickels K, Geller AM. Chronic use of benzodiazepines and psychomotor and cognitive test performance. *Psychopharmacology* 1986; **88**: 426-33.
(17) Mellinger GD, Balter MB. Prevalence and patterns of use of psychotherapeutic drugs: Results from a 1979 national survey of American adults. In: Tognoni G, Ballantuono C, Lader M, eds. *Epidemiologic impact of psychotropic drugs*. Amsterdam: Elsevier North Holland, 1981: 117-35.

Discussion

Dr File said that studies of tolerance had shown just as marked an episodic anterograde amnesia in highly anxious patients as in normal volunteers. Whereas for tasks that depended on speed an anxious patient might improve while on benzodiazepines, the amnesia remained as great. Two separate factors led to prolonged use of certain benzodiazepines. One was the severity of the withdrawal reaction, which may be related to the half-life. The other, the extent to which patients liked individual benzodiazepines (and they were not all liked equally). This was important, and was echoed in the black market price, which was not the same for all benzodiazepines. Rats also seemed to find some compounds pleasant and others less so, and remarkably, they echoed the human taste preferences.

Dr Tyrer wondered whether the problems that arose with short-acting benzodiazepines could be explained in pharmacokinetic terms, or whether they could be related to other factors, such as the potency of the compounds. Most of the short-acting compounds were more potent than the long-acting ones, and the receptor affinity played a part there. This was an important point from the pharmaceutical industry's viewpoint, because there was a trend towards shorter and shorter-acting benzodiazepines, but if such compounds conferred greater risks, their development ought to be halted.

Dr Wheatley thought that the reason for the initial prescription of benzodiazepines was important, when considering comparisons between short- and long-acting compounds. Many anxiolytics were prescribed for a situational anxiety, which occurred perhaps at one time in the day only, where a short-acting compound would be appropriate. To prescribe a long-acting drug for a situation which recurred daily would lead eventually to a steady state plasma level. One of his patients had to attend a conference each morning, where she felt a great deal of pressure and responsibility, and took temazepam, which had been prescribed to help her sleep; it did not make her sleep, but it prevented her panic, and she took it each morning and not at weekends. This seemed to be a useful drug regime for that particular case, and in prescribing short-acting drugs, their indications for use as well as possible potential for dependence should be considered.

Dr Beary said that speed of onset was also important. His own research had shown a measured effect on the adrenal cortical system within 40 min of oral ingestion of the drug. He also pointed out that temazepam was marketed in Italy as a day-time anxiolytic.

Adjustment disorders and environmental change — benzodiazepines and other treatments in general practice

ROGER HIGGS

Department of General Practice Studies, King's College School of Medicine and Dentistry, Denmark Hill, London SE5 9RS, UK

The presentations of psychological distress to general practice are extremely varied, and may not be well understood if the starting point is symptomatology; before a major psychiatric illness emerges, 'minor disorders' may present either with physical symptoms or a mixture of physical and psychological complaints. The current research position is well summarized by Clare and Blacker (1). Multi-axial classification is a necessity, and the question in general practice is not so much 'What is psychiatric?' but in each presentation, 'How much is psychiatric?' Follow-up studies indicate that a large proportion of patients get better, but up to a third may remain unwell when assessed within the year of initial presentation (2).

Studies of doctors' behaviour and of illness behaviour in patients establish that many other factors determine the decision to seek medical help (3). Thus, a model emerges of a vulnerable person at risk or facing a crisis whose coping mechanisms fail, and who develops a physical or psychological feeling which has a worrying association or meaning.

Studies show that the patient is often at a point of particular stress because he/she is attempting to adjust to a necessary or anticipated change in living or perception of living (4,5). The examination of these psychosocial transitions and the disorders of adjustment that arise from them may give a better understanding of minor disorders than concentration on symptomatology.

The work currently available (much of it descriptive) makes it clear that patients often present to primary care doctors at a period of environmental or personal change, which is related to life events. The work of Brown *et al.* (6) is well known, and this approach has been pursued in general practice in such studies as that by Ingham and Miller (7), who found that over a third of patients who had recently consulted their doctors reported either major threatening life events or difficulties in the recent past. Such changes may be more difficult to pin down in two ways (8). Firstly, the event that is used as the index in such a study or in the surgery may have a superficial, symbolic, or paradoxical relationship to the transition which is in progress. The event which has caused a reaction may appear to be a minor one to the observer, but may be

The benzodiazepines in current clinical practice, edited by Hugh Freeman and Yvonne Rue, 1987: Royal Society of Medicine Services International Congress and Symposium Series No. 114, published by Royal Society of Medicine Services Limited.

'the last straw' or the crucial event by which the individual recognizes that this is a time of crisis. Equally, a small or apparently unrelated event may suddenly bring to the mind of the patient his condition—such as when, following a bereavement with which the patient has coped well, there is a sudden realization that something which had been dealt with together now has to be faced alone. A paradoxical event to the observer is one that apparently implies progress or satisfaction, but may have caused a loss elsewhere in the person's life. There is an additional difficulty in that most life event inventories deal with recent life events, but research on occurrences further into the past makes it clear that the psychological 'fuse' for these events may be long and slow. It is the *meaning* that they provide for the patient which is crucial, both to the presentation and to the type of therapy that can be applied. In this context, it is personal calendar time (anniversaries), biological time (such as the 40th birthday), or psychic time that may be the most important.

Not enough study has been done of major or minor illness as a life event in itself, or as the creator of an environment in which the patient comes to recognize and therefore to accept or to resist psycho-social changes. While the illness is of greatest importance to the doctor, this may not be the case for the patient, and therefore should not necessarily be so for the research worker. A natural concern with pathology blinds us to the fact that this is an area where there is literally a growth industry. Any form of preventive or anticipatory care in general practice has to help the patient face change in a positive way, and must assess the growth and progress which may be made even in the face of physical decline (9). It is sad that the therapies currently applied have been so often driven to the edges of accepted practice by mainstream clinical work, but encouraging to see some problem-solving approaches in psychiatric practice attempting to redress this balance. Management strategies depend as much on helping the patient to see the potential for a positive outcome, while making sense of the current episode, as they are concerned with symptomatology. Seen in terms of prognosis, follow-up studies of 'minor' affective disorders reveal a group in which the crisis may be productive, a second group who are developing a major disorder, and a third group of chronically malfunctioning people in whom things have become worse. In the last of these, all treatment schedules must be considered potentially long-term, and the dangers of dependency should be considered (10,11,12). In the first group, however, the necessity for medication in the treatment of symptoms must depend on the value to the patient of the symptom at the time. If the symptom is in some senses 'useful' to enable the patient to make a realistic adjustment, the balance and logic of prescribing, as well as prescribing in conjunction with other therapies, must be carefully considered.

References

(1) Clare AW, Blacker R. Some problems affecting the diagnosis and classification of depressive disorders in primary care. In: Shepherd M, Wilkinson G, Williams P, eds. *Mental illness in primary care setting*. London: Tavistock Publications, 1986: 7–26.
(2) Wilkinson G. *Overview of mental health practices in primary care settings, with recommendations for further research*. Washington DC: National Institute of Mental Health, 1986.
(3) Tuckett D. Becoming a patient. In: Tuckett D, ed. *An introduction to medical sociology*. London: Tavistock Publications, 1976: 159–89.
(4) Parkes CM. Psychosocial transitions: a field for study. *Soc Sci Med* 1971; **5**: 101–15.
(5) Higgs R. Life changes. *Br Med J* 1984; **288**: 1556–7.

(6) Brown GW, Harris T. *Social origins of depression*. London: Tavistock Publications, 1978.
(7) Ingham J, Miller P. Symptom prevalence and severity in a general practice population. *J Epidemiol Comm Hlth* 1979; **33**: 191-8.
(8) Higgs R. *Psychosocial problems 1-4*. Postgraduate Partwork Series. Horton Kirby: Modern Medicine Publications, 1983.
(9) Royal College of General Practitioners. *Prevention of psychiatric disorders in general practice*. Report from general practice no. 20. London: Royal College of General Practitioners, 1981.
(10) Catalan J, Gaff DH. Benzodiazepines in general practice: time for a decision. *Br Med J* 1985; **290**: 1374-6.
(11) Jones L, Simpson D, Brown A, Bainton D, McDonald H. Prescribing psychotropic drugs in general practice: a three-year study. *Br Med J* 1984; **289**: 1045-8.
(12) Catalan J, Gaff G, Edmonds G, Bond A, Martin P, Ennis J. The effects of non-prescribing of anxiolytics in general practice. *Br J Psych* 1984; **144**: 593-610.

Benzodiazepines and the general physician

PAUL TURNER

*Department of Clinical Pharmacology,
St Bartholomew's Hospital, London EC1A 7BE*

Major interest in the use and abuse of benzodiazepines has centred around their administration for treatment of anxiety states and as hypnotics; like general practitioners and psychiatrists, general physicians and other hospital clinicians use them widely for these purposes.

A recent study in St Bartholomew's Hospital, London (1) showed that 42% of a sample of general surgical in-patients and 40% of a sample of general medical in-patients had been prescribed benzodiazepines: of these prescriptions, 85% were as hypnotics and 15% for their anxiolytic effects. Almost all the prescriptions for hypnotics were on an as-required basis, few patients actually requesting or receiving them, while the prescriptions for their anxiolytic use were generally for regular administration. However, a survey carried out at the same time of prescriptions for medical and surgical patients on discharge showed that only 4·8% were continuing to take benzodiazepines when they left hospital. This limited local experience in a London teaching hospital with district responsibilities does not suggest, therefore, that use of benzodiazepines as hypnotics and anxiolytics represents an important initiating source of long-term use and abuse. Some evidence for increasing restraint in the prescription of hypnotic drugs is seen in comparing these recent prescribing figures with those obtained in the same hospital in a survey of drug prescribing in January 1971, when 60% of in-patients were prescribed hypnotics. Furthermore, the prescription of an as-required benzodiazepine is a legitimate and convenient practice for patients who are distressed by insomnia because of the noisy environment of a busy ward, or by the apprehension and anxiety of their condition.

Although these indications may account numerically for the majority of prescriptions for benzodiazepines in general medical and surgical wards, as well as in general practice and psychiatry, doctors working in certain special hospital departments find that they are of value in a much wider range of clinical indications, and these must be considered in any recommendations made about their use in hospital medicine.

A list of clinical indications which have been claimed to be appropriate for benzodiazepine treatment is given in Table 1. Not all clinicians would agree on their value in all of these conditions, while in some, such as eclampsia, there are marked international differences in treatment practice. Nevertheless, they are widely used in

---

The benzodiazepines in current clinical practice, edited by Hugh Freeman and Yvonne Rue, 1987: Royal Society of Medicine Services International Congress and Symposium Series No. 114, published by Royal Society of Medicine Services Limited.

Table 1
Some clinical indications which have been claimed to be appropriate for benzodiazepine treatment

Psychiatric	Hypnotic
	Anxiety
	Tardive dyskinesias, dystonias
	Alcohol/drug withdrawal reactions
	Night terrors and somnambulism
Neurological	Epilepsy, febrile seizures
	Spasticity
	Spasmodic torticollis
	Migraine prophylaxis
	Vertigo
Gastrointestinal	Irritable bowel syndrome
Obstetric	Eclampsia, pre-eclampsia
Anaesthetic/surgical	Operative premedication, general and local anaesthesia
	Endoscopy
	Induction
	Neuroleptanalgesia
	Intensive care
Dermatology	Oral lichen planus
General	Potentiation of analgesics

these conditions, and in some they represent a considerable advance on their predecessors — particularly the barbiturates, which had marked respiratory-depressant and dependence-producing properties.

Psychiatric

General physicians and non-psychiatric specialties often have patients with psychiatric problems which require treatment. The value of benzodiazepines as hypnotics, anxiolytics, and in the management of patients with alcohol and other drug withdrawal reactions is well established, although because the latter often abuse multiple drugs including benzodiazepines, these preparations should only be used when clearly indicated and for the minimum time required (2). Their use in tardive dyskinesia and in paediatric sleep disorders such as night terrors and somnambulism is less well established, although some individual patients may be helped by them (3).

Neurological

The use of intravenous diazepam and clonazepam in treatment of status epilepticus and febrile seizures is now well established, but their oral use, and that of clobazam for maintenance prophylactic treatment is still being evaluated (4,5). Diazepam is of value in some patients with spasticity associated with multiple sclerosis and other spinal cord disease, although sedation may limit its use. Benzodiazepines are sometimes used in patients with migraine (3) or vertigo (6) in whom anxiety is prominent and may precipitate or aggravate their symptoms, but they cannot be considered a satisfactory or specific form of treatment for these conditions.

Gastrointestinal

Treatment of the ill-defined irritable bowel syndrome is unsatisfactory, as is demonstrated by the many forms of dietary and drug regimes which have been used in its management. Benzodiazepines have been claimed to be of value in some patients, but should be restricted to those who fail to respond to other measures, and only be used in short courses (3).

Obstetric

Diazepam is considered in this country to be among the first drugs of choice for patients with pre-eclampsia or eclampsia (7), while in North America magnesium sulphate is primarily recommended (8).

Anaesthetic, surgical, intensive care

The importance of allaying anxiety in patients with life-threatening conditions, in intensive care, preoperatively, or before and during endoscopy, cardiac catheterization, and other invasive diagnostic procedures cannot be over-emphasized, and it would be negligent to withhold benzodiazepines for such indications because of fear of abuse. Furthermore, they have amnesic properties which are of particular value when they are used to sedate patients for minor but unpleasant diagnostic and surgical procedures which may need to be repeated on several occasions.

The large increase in number of day-case procedures carried out in hospitals over recent years owes much to the introduction of short-acting benzodiazepines, such as intravenous midazolam, which produce sub-anaesthetic effects of sedation plus amnesia, and is therefore a valuable premedicant in these situations (9).

Dermatological

Some skin conditions such as lichen planus, which can become widespread, erosive and ulcerative, appear to be precipitated or aggravated by emotional factors, and anxiolytic treatment with benzodiazepines may be of value in these (3).

The elderly patient

Care of elderly patients continues to be, and is becoming increasingly the responsibility of general physicians, very often for social as well as for strictly clinical indications. A considerable number of such patients are already taking benzodiazepines when admitted. Trewin et al. (10) found that 18·7% of 1260 admissions to a geriatric unit were taking benzodiazepine hypnotics, of which 40% were nitrazepam and 43% temazepam. Prescriptions for 53·8% of these patients were discontinued after admission, but 31·8% had them continued throughout the admission and were prescribed a further supply as take-home medication. Of all the admissions 8·6% were newly prescribed a benzodiazepine hypnotic in hospital, and about one-quarter of these continued to take it following discharge. If this experience in Exeter is not unrepresentative of the situation elsewhere in the United Kingdom, it confirms the widespread view that many elderly patients in the community are being prescribed these drugs on a long-term basis unnecessarily, and that they could successfully be weaned off them. The number needing to take them after discharge (8·2% of the total number of patients admitted) was not unexpected, however, in a population of elderly patients who had required admission for a variety of both social and pathological conditions, and is not very different from the 4·8% found in our own recent survey of general medical and surgical discharges from a general hospital which included many elderly patients.

Conclusions

Most of the indications in Table 1 only involve relatively short-term administration, either single doses or over a few days, and are unlikely to produce problems of dependence or abuse. Some, however, including epilepsy and chronic neurological disorders such as spasticity, may require longer-term treatment. In these cases, the possible dangers of abuse and dependence will require a risk-benefit judgment to be made for each patient on the basis of the severity of their condition, and their history and personality. However, in these particular indications, most alternative forms of treatment have potential adverse effects which are less tolerable or more serious than those of the benzodiazepines.

Benzodiazepines have proved to be effective and valuable drugs for a wide range of indications in hospital in-patients, day-case patients, and out-patient referrals. The increased sensitivity of elderly patients to their effects should be reflected in careful choice of the prescribed dosage and of the duration of treatment (3). Their appropriate and careful use should not be associated with dependence or abuse on a significant scale.

References

(1) Holland A, Turner P. Personal communication.
(2) Peachey JE, Naranjo CA. The role of drugs in the treatment of alcoholism. *Drugs* 1984; **27**: 171–82.
(3) Avery GS. *Drug treatment*, 2nd ed. Edinburgh: Churchill Livingstone, 1980.
(4) Eadie MJ, Tyrer JH. *Anticonvulsant therapy: pharmacological basis and practice*, 2nd ed. Edinburgh: Churchill Livingstone, 1980.
(5) Beghi E, Di Mascio A, Tognoni G. Drug treatment of epilepsy. *Drugs* 1986; **31**: 249–65.
(6) Oosterveld WJ. Vertigo: current concepts in management. *Drugs* 1985; **30**: 275–83.
(7) Lewis PJ. *Therapeutic problems in pregnancy*. Lancaster: MTP Press, 1977.
(8) Rayburn WF, Zuspan FP. *Drug therapy in obstetrics and gynaecology*. Norwalk, Conn: Appleton-Century-Crofts, 1982.
(9) Dundee JW, Halliday NJ, Hasper KW, Brogden RN. Midazolam: a review of its pharmacological properties and therapeutic use. *Drugs* 1984; **28**: 519–43.
(10) Trewin VF, Pearce V, Veitch GBA. Elderly patients at risk. *Br J Pharm Pract* 1986; **8**: 359–63.

Discussion

Dr Wheatley wished to add one important indication to the list—that of pre-menstrual syndrome (PMS); this is a common condition, which varies considerably in its symptomatology and duration, but anxiety and particularly depressive symptoms are usually a feature. Antidepressants are not indicated here, however, because the condition does not last longer than 14 days at any one time, which is the time taken for an antidepressant to exert any marked effect. It represents a clear indication for using a benzodiazepine, preferably one with antidepressant properties such as alprazolam; the medication is very effective, and the patient would be off it for two weeks or more, because symptoms are often maximal only three or four days before a period. This is a self-limiting disease, which needs control because of its sometimes unfortunate consequences, and represents an important non-psychiatric indication for the use of a benzodiazepine, but only when anxiety and/or depressive symptoms are prominent.

Professor Clare said that there were a large number of conditions where current treatments were not very effective, and it was therefore not surprising that a non-specific, general, all-purpose drug—the benzodiazepines was widely used. A study at St Bartholomew's Hospital in 1987 was finding that, as distinct from the 1960s, PMS was hard to find, since it was heavily contaminated with other disorders, from adjustment problems to the classical anxiety state. It was also extremely sensitive on a temporary basis to a wide variety of interventions, from aldosterone to vitamin B6, but what was most interesting was that many women resisted the idea of using benzodiazepines. He did not altogether agree with some of the more enthusiastic comments that had been made with regard to the use of benzodiazepines in such non-specific conditions, but accepted that these conditions were difficult to diagnose, manage, and treat. It was surprising that in the field of PMS, not one single study in the literature had followed patients for longer than a year, and there was no indication as to what happened to those people at the end of that time. In the cases of PMS, irritable bowel syndrome, and migraine prophylaxis, benzodiazepines should be used with considerable caution. On the other hand, cognitive therapists or behavioural counsellors could be effective in the treatment of PMS; the numbers of patients are small, they are highly motivated, and there is good evidence that they respond to behavioural treatment of a non-physical kind.

Dr Tyrer raised the question of adjustment disorders as a description. It was a diagnosis related to life events, and allowed mixed symptoms—the only diagnosis, in fact, which allowed mixed affective symptoms to occur together. But precise information about it was lacking. It had been said earlier that too much attention was paid to symptoms and not enough to life events, and that patients going into hospital for general medical and surgical problems could be described as having anxieties such as adjustment disorders. Perhaps in these situations the benzodiazepines were being used properly, but there was a deficiency of formal studies about them.

Referring to Dr Higgs' presentation, **Dr Marks** said that patients often showed the 'clothes-peg phenomenon'—attaching a label onto an internal sense of autonomic over-activity. He agreed that internal, personal, psychological, and family factors were important, but felt that wider social factors were also worth considering. In the Edinburgh area, he had not seen the number of agoraphobics and phobics that he saw in the estates around Liverpool: it had been suggested that Scotsmen found such phobias unacceptable and so the women in the population did not develop them with any great frequency.

Dr Higgs found it fascinating that a general practitioner became closely allied to the methods and thoughts of his patients: he had to look at things the way the patients did. In his own area, the fear of assault was now so high that many people who would otherwise go out and find their own way of dealing with problems were staying in their houses; even among 17–18 year old men, there was fear of attack, although it was not clear whether or not they were right about this. In general practice, the doctor had to find both the social reasons for illness and the social treatments to fit particular patients. A recent study in his practice of psychosocial stresses or concerns of patients had found that men in the inner city had a far greater number of worries than men elsewhere about their debts, their marriages, or their housing conditions. How one dealt with such problems was related more to how the patient perceived them than how they actually were.

Part of the key to his method of treatment was to allow the patient to use these drugs as she felt most appropriate. The question of the number of prescriptions written as opposed to the number cashed reminded him of a general practice with a large yew tree in the car park. When this tree was cut down it was found to be full of prescription forms which the patients had stuffed into the trunk as they went out. Many of the people suffering adjustment disorders used only a small number of the tablets that were prescribed, simply to get over the particular crisis, and in such a situation prescribing was often symbolic. It meant that someone was taking notice of the patient and would give help if it was needed.

Professor Clare thought that this comment might hold the key to some of the prescribing in general practice. Two thousand attenders at a north London practice had recently been studied by Blacker and himself, and the main purpose had been to establish the prevalence, nature, course and outcome of severe depressive illness; the SADS interview and the PSE had been used to generate a variety of diagnostic categories. They had also looked at the extent to which the features of the illness and its diagnostic categories were changed by altering the instruments used. The overall prevalence of psychiatric disorder was 35·5%; adjustment disorder, using the criteria given by Dr Higgs, accounted for about 50% — a figure that had been unexpected.

Some diagnostic framework was needed to bring general practitioners and specialists closer together: the term 'mixed minor affective disorder' was not very helpful from the GP's point of view, although it described what the psychiatrist saw in that setting, and the classification of these groups of disorder was still debatable. He did not think it could necessarily be said that adjustment disorder was a condition for which benzodiazepines should be prescribed.

Professor Rickels said that there had been few controlled studies in such disorders and that they were difficult to investigate because the course was so short that precise measurements were hard to take. Nevertheless, if he could alleviate some suffering for a patient for two or three days, it was right to do so. In a generalized anxiety disorder, the use of benzodiazepines is indicated on a temporary, limited, and clearly proscribed basis. An example of a situation where temporary medication should be given for adjustment stress was a woman in her late 30s who suddenly developed a lump in her breast and had to go for a biopsy some days later; she became very anxious and could not sleep. In this stress situation, where the resolution is swift, temporary use of benzodiazepines was appropriate.

Professor Clare concluded that there was agreement that relief in the short-term for general medical disorders was a legitimate use of the drug.

Professor Lader returned to the symbolic nature of the prescription, since problems arose with the need to prescribe for other than medical reasons. Many patients had adjustment reactions, and the Oxford study (Catalan J, Gath D, Edmonds G, Ennis J. *Br J Psych* 1984; **144**: 593–602) had shown that this group responded well to non-pharmacological means. However, symptomatic relief for three or four days was not the only element of the equation: other factors included prescribing for reasons not clearly defined, the knowledge that other forms of treatment might be at least as effective, and the unknown problems of how many people would continue the medication because they liked its effect upon them. Most importantly, how many people would be taught by that first attendance and prescription that the next time they had a problem in adjusting to life events, they could simply take medication? He believed that symptomatic relief was only a relatively small factor; it was also important to train patients to deal with their problems without resorting to medication.

Professor Clare asked why there was no evidence of chronic use in young patients; why did they stop, and not turn to benzodiazepines every time there was a crisis?

Dr Williams said that this had not been specifically studied, but he suspected that if it was, most people would say that they stopped because they felt better — in other words it had got them through their acute situational crisis. One further point with regard to the symbolic function of a prescription was that it might not be necessary for potent medicine to be prescribed for this purpose, but rather a placebo. If a pharmacologically impotent substance could fulfil this purpose, perhaps that was something that should be considered, though it raised interesting ethical issues.

Dr Higgs was unsure of the value of placebos, because he felt that his aim was to help the patient to understand their situation, and to give them the tools to deal with it. Most young people knew that the crisis was short-term, and just wanted to get through it; they could not take time off work at that stage to meet a cognitive therapist, and in general they resolved the problems themselves. What was much more difficult was the chronically dissatisfied, unhappy 40 year-old who depended on the regular pill, and older people who suffered from sleeplessness. These situations presented the problem of a continued behaviour pattern.

Dr Imlah commented that people who used alcohol were not remaining substance-free — they were instead using a substance that was easily obtainable in the community. Although they did not take drugs, they solved their problems with other forms of relief. However, there is widespread consumption of benzodiazepines among narcotic users: a high proportion of people on methodone maintenance are also taking them, and the most popular in Birmingham is temazepam for daytime use. In New Zealand, where illicit drugs are less easy to obtain, there is a great problem with flunitrazepam.

Dr Beary referred to the suggestion that benzodiazepines are not prescribed to the young: in fact, 40% of benzodiazepines are prescribed for those under 40, and people in their 20s are given benzodiazepines quite commonly by their general practitioners. Professor Clare had asked why were there not considerable numbers of chronic users among the young, but this was a different question. Although drug addicts largely take benzodiazepines for the abuse effect rather than to relieve symptoms, there is a cross-over effect, and they obtain their drugs from general practitioners because it is so easy to do so.

Professor Freeman raised the subject of neuroses developing after accidents, where it could be argued that more benzodiazepines ought to be used, rather than less. People with prolonged disability following accidents had generally suffered very severe anxiety and terror in the period immediately after the event. This had lasted for perhaps a week, and in most cases they had had no relief at all, whereas it is likely that effective treatment of that anxiety initially might have spared many of them the prolonged disability that they subsequently suffered.

Professor Lader agreed, and compared that to the shell shock syndrome. In the First World War, its victims were not treated, and not many of them returned to battle, but in the Second they were treated with barbiturates, and after about two weeks of intensive sedation, many went back into action.

Mr Taylor regretted that the pharmaceutical industry was not in a position to give precise information as to who took benzodiazepines, for how long, and what the relevant problems were. There had been debates for over 15 years on this subject, but still the work necessary to elucidate its various aspects had not been done. However, in relation to illegal drug use, he was not sure whether the benzodiazepines were causal. When a condition generated unpleasant feelings for which the drug wanted was not available, it was natural to turn to another drug to control the bad feelings until the preparation desired was available.

Dr Wells said it was generally accepted that the benzodiazepines were extremely useful, but both the industry and doctors were attacked because of the unpleasant, long-term effects which people experienced after using them. Further consideration was needed of how to get the right message across to doctors who were not using benzodiazepines appropriately in their prescribing.

Professor Lader said that if all Dr Wells' patients came off benzodiazepines by four months, this could be done by all general practitioners. The problem was the small proportion of GPs who were not doing that, and who were in fact doing badly by their patients. However, **Professor Clare** believed it was not absolutely clear what guidelines should be given to GPs at the present time. There had been considerable confusion during the past five years over the definition of short-acting and long-acting compounds respectively. There was also the question of whether long-term use led to escalation, and if not, should benzodiazepines be bought over the counter. It was not only GPs but also the specialists who were not absolutely at one about the guidelines.

Long-term benzodiazepine use and psychological functioning

MALCOLM LADER

*Department of Psychiatry, Institute of Psychiatry,
De Crespigny Park, London SE5 8AF, UK*

The benzodiazepines provide the main drug treatment of patients with generalized anxiety disorder, and despite increasing knowledge of problems attending their use—both short-term and long-term—they remain popular; indeed, their consumption in the USA is increasing, mainly due to the success of alprazolam. In 1981, a survey of the adult population of the UK revealed that 11·6% had taken some tranquillizer/sedative type of medication on one or more days during the preceding 12 months (1). This figure was further broken down into 4·2% who had used for less than one month, 2·5% for 1-3 months, 0·8% for 4-11 months, and 3·1% for 12 months or more, i.e. continuously; the latter represents about a million and a quarter adults.

However, little is known of either the benefits or the drawbacks associated with long-term benzodiazepine use. Many studies have evaluated their efficacy in various indications, including the anxiety disorders, while others have quantified the psychological effects of these drugs, either given in single doses or as short courses of treatment. But the methodological problems of studying the long-term use of benzodiazepines has precluded any precise assessment of either long-term efficacy or unwanted effects.

This contribution will briefly review what is known of the psychological effects of long-term benzodiazepine treatment, concentrating on psychomotor, cognitive, and memory functions.

Problem of method

The problems of method can be divided into three main groups—those associated with the practicalities of assessing various aspects of psychological functioning, those related to pharmacological factors, and those related to the design of studies and choice of subjects.

Very large numbers of tests are available. Hindmarch (2) lists the following: proof reading ability, spiral after-effect duration, low-speed car handling tasks, card sorting ability, car driving simulator, pursuit rotor, symbol copying, absolute auditory

The benzodiazepines in current clinical practice, edited by Hugh Freeman and Yvonne Rue, 1987: Royal Society of Medicine Services International Congress and Symposium Series No. 114, published by Royal Society of Medicine Services Limited.

threshold, short- and long-term memory, verbal learning, discrimination conditioning of the eyelid response, kinaesthetic figural after-effect, muscular grip strength, adaptive tracking, beam balancing task, digit symbol substitution task, delayed auditory feedback, ocular convergence, the speed of putting caps on ballpoint pens, tapping speed, hidden word task, auditory reaction time, Gibson spiral maze, critical flicker fusion frequency, time estimation procedure, digit span test, response time, body sway, duration of after-images, serial subtraction of numbers, Purdue pegboard, stabilometer, concentration, concept identification task, group vigilance task, cancellation of numbers, category clustering, saccadic eye movements, rudder control test, choice reaction time task, car driving ability, spontaneous reversals of the Necker cube, two-handed coordination, Whipple's tracing board and a trigram recognition task. This list is by no means exhaustive, however.

A wide range of functions can be tested, and are roughly subsumed under the following headings: sensory function and sensory processing ability; CNS function and central processing ability including memory and learning; motor function and behavioural coordination; sensorimotor performance. Psychomotor performance is the outcome of coordinated sensory and motor systems through the integrative and organizational activities of the brain, while personality, memory and motivation influence the processing of sensory information. The coordinated behavioural responses are themselves modified by adaptive and feedback mechanisms.

Motivational factors can alter performance. These include the expectations of both experimenter and subjects, the level of payment, and the context in which the study is conducted. Double-blind procedures, careful screening of volunteers, well-trained experimenters, and strict adherence to a carefully constructed protocol are therefore essential.

Tests involving the coordination of sensory and motor system functions can show practice effects. One approach is to test every subject repeatedly until they reach a plateau performance, but this can be very tedious, as improvement in performance can continue over many repetitions of the test. Other tests may need the use of parallel versions to prevent the subject becoming familiar with their content.

The pharmacological factors which complicate the issue are those of accumulation, tolerance, and withdrawal. Accumulation is a predictable phenomenon, depending on the elimination half-life of the benzodiazepine; anxiolytic benzodiazepines are divisible into the medium and long-acting groups; hypnotics also have short-acting types (Table 1). The long-acting drugs will certainly accumulate, and the medium-acting may do so to some extent, but more markedly in the elderly. If effects on psychological functioning are related to bodily concentrations, then impairments should increase during the phase of accumulation, i.e. over about four times the elimination half-life of the compound or of any active metabolites.

A countervailing influence is that of tolerance. Rickels *et al.* (3,4) have adduced evidence that the anti-anxiety effects of benzodiazepines are maintained for up to 22 weeks, i.e. that tolerance does not occur. Tolerance also failed to supervene to reduction in critical flicker fusion thresholds or impairment of short-term memory (5). However, subjective sedation and psychomotor impairment does show tolerance to continuing benzodiazepine use (6,7).

The third pharmacological factor is withdrawal (8). Discontinuation of medication is often followed by rebound, varying in degree from minor discomfort—anxiety, insomnia and tension—to a major syndrome (9). Attempts to test subjects during the withdrawal phase will be confounded by the increases in anxiety.

It is also important to differentiate between reversible drug-related impairments and irreversible deficits, which perhaps reflect neuronal damage. Alcohol abuse

Table 1
Some anxiolytic and hypnotic benzodiazepines

Anxiolytics	Absorption rate	Duration of clinical effect	Sedative effects	Accumulation	Withdrawal problems
Long-acting					
Chlordiazepoxide	Rapid	Long	Minor	Marked	Minor
Diazepam	Rapid	Long	Minor	Marked	Marked
Medium-acting					
Oxazepam	Slow	Intermediate	Minor	Minor	Minor
Lorazepam	Intermediate	Intermediate	Marked	Minor	Marked

Hypnotics	Absorption rate	Duration of clinical effect	Residual effects	Accumulation	Rebound effects
Long-acting					
Nitrazepam	Intermediate	Long	Marked	Marked	Minor
Medium-acting					
Temazepam	Slow	Intermediate	Minor	Minor	Minor
Short-acting					
Triazolam	Rapid	Short	Minimal	Nil	Marked

provides the best-documented example of this, but there is evidence that even moderate drinking may be associated with deterioration in psychological functioning (10).

Problems of study design concern differences between normal subjects and anxious patients, single-dose and repeated dose administration, short-term and long-term treatment, and therapeutic doses compared with high-dose abuse. These differences with respect to benzodiazepine effects will now be outlined.

Anxiety and psychological functioning

Of itself, anxiety affects psychological functioning, with quite marked impairments being found on some measures. For example, we compared 30 drug-free patients suffering from chronic anxiety disorders with 30 normal controls matched for age, sex, and social class (11). Card-sorting into categories and simple piles, digit symbol substitution tests, symbol copying, simple arithmetic, and tachistoscopic recognition were all significantly impaired in the patients; however, auditory reaction time, simple tapping, Gibson spiral maze, and cancellation tests were not affected. We concluded that as task complexity increased, patient performance was more impaired.

An implication of this finding is that treatments which lower anxiety will tend to improve performance indirectly, which nullifies any direct depressant effect of the medication. Those direct effects are consequently better studied in normal subjects, at least initially in the programme of research; armed with this knowledge, the researcher can then better interpret his data from patients. Empirically, it is important to establish whether patients are psychologically impaired while on benzodiazepines (12). Dosage is crucial: a high dose will produce impairment in patients, but what is more important is to see whether impairment supervenes at clinically effective doses.

Single-doses in normals

A large literature has accrued concerning the effects of single doses of anxiolytics and hypnotics on a variety of tests. For example, Johnson and Chernik (13) reviewed 52 studies, mostly involving single doses of hypnotics in normal subjects; they listed the tests used and the proportion of investigations in which each test was sensitive to benzodiazepine effects. Card sorting was most useful in discriminating between hypnotic/sedative and placebo, with 11 out of 18 test comparisons (61%) being positive. Symbol copying, tapping rate, digit symbol substitution, memory, arithmetic, and vigilance tasks were all discriminatory in a third or more of studies, while coordination tasks, critical flicker fusion, pursuit rotor, Purdue pegboard, and simple or choice reaction times were least useful. It thus seemed that the speed at which simple acts of a repetitive nature are performed is most likely to be impaired by benzodiazepines, especially where the motor component is linked to a learning or memory component.

Repeated doses in normals

The most commonly used tests are reaction time, digit symbol substitution, cancellation, tapping, card sorting, pursuit rotor, and critical flicker fusion. The most sensitive, i.e. those which have discriminated most significantly between a benzodiazepine and a placebo, are critical flicker fusion, learning and memory, digit symbol substitution, cancellation, and card sorting (2). Relatively insensitive functions are complex visual motor coordination, visual spatial performance, and auditory perception. Also, benzodiazepines have little effect on such established functions as visual-spatial, perceptual, and verbal tasks, whereas the acquisition of new material, as sampled by memory functions and digit symbol substitution, is sensitive to these drugs. Speed of repetitive movements such as tapping, cancellation, and card sorting is relatively sensitive to drug effects. The discrepancies between tests sensitive to single doses and those sensitive to repeated doses are most easily explained in terms of tolerance.

Short-term effects in patients

Several years ago, we demonstrated the difficulty in detecting any effects of benzodiazepines given for a few weeks on psychological functioning in anxious patients (14). Tranquillization improves performance because it counteracts the disruptive effect of the anxiety disorder. Similar conclusions were obtained in a study of the residual effects of hypnotics in a sample of 60 severely anxious in-patients (15): card sorting and Gibson spiral maze time were marginally affected after a week of treatment with N-desmethyldiazepam, 20 mg at night.

Over the short-term, then, the symptomatic relief afforded by the benzodiazepines also tends to improve psychological functioning, provided the dose level is judiciously chosen. Under-dosage will be associated with failure to improve, and too high a dose will push the patient over the top of the classical inverted U-shaped curve, resulting in definite impairment.

Long-term effects in patients

The situation becomes even more complex over the longer term. Cumulation of longer-acting benzodiazepines is inevitable and, unless counteracted by tissue tolerance, would lead to gross impairment. But remission of the anxiety disorder will also complicate the issue: if the anxiety lessens, then anxiety-related performance decrements will also lessen, and the benzodiazepine is much more likely to result in psychological impairments. Of course, patients in remission would be expected to discontinue their benzodiazepine consumption, although some patients may develop normal dose dependence and continue their medication indefinitely.

Our own interest in the long-term effects of benzodiazepines on psychological performance was stimulated by a pilot study in 22 patients withdrawing from normal-dose long-term benzodiazepine treatment; their data were compared with those of two control groups — one recruited from research and technical staff, the other from the community. Both patients and controls were assessed repeatedly on the digit symbol substitution test, symbol copying test, cancellation task, auditory reaction time, and key tapping rate; a substantial and prolonged practice effect was found on all the tests except reaction time and key-tapping. Prior to withdrawal, the patients did not show the performance decrement on the cancellation task, reaction time, and key tapping which is customarily associated with the initial phases of benzodiazepine therapy. However, a rebound performance increment was observed on tapping rate during the withdrawal: patients demonstrated impaired performance on tasks requiring the combined use of sensory and fine motor skills (16).

The only entirely rigorous way of assessing the long-term effects of benzodiazepines is by prospective random allocation of newly-presenting patients with acute generalized anxiety disorders to treatment with either placebo or a benzodiazepine. Those patients in whom long-term treatment can be justified ethically would be tested at appropriate time-points. Because the indications for long-term use are limited and because worries about dependence are increasing, the proportion of anxious patients commencing anti-anxiety medication going on to long-term use is tending to diminish. Consequently, a very large cohort would have to start treatment in order to end up with adequate numbers at the one-year time-point. Yet many long-term users have been on benzodiazepines for a decade or more, and are the subject of particular concern. Even if the substantial financial resources for a large-scale study became available, we cannot wait until the turn of the century before being able to make recommendations regarding the advisability of prolonged treatment. A parallel situation has existed for almost 20 years with antipsychotic medication and the risk of tardive dyskinesia, yet practical guidelines for medication can be drawn up, despite major areas of continuing ignorance.

Thus, to make any immediate progress, a cross-sectional study has to be resorted to, despite the obvious limitations. To that end, my research team has been involved in an extensive study to evaluate the psychological effects of long-term benzodiazepine therapy (17); my co-workers were Dr Susan Golombok, a psychologist, and Dr Parimala Moodley, a psychiatrist.

Major practical problems were encountered in obtaining appropriate patients who met our strict criteria, but 145 subjects were tested. They comprised three groups: patients currently taking benzodiazepines; patients who had stopped taking benzodiazepines; and subjects who had never taken benzodiazepines or who had done so in the past for less than one year. Those currently on benzodiazepines ($n=50$) were identified through the records of several general practitioners in the London area. The criterion for inclusion was the taking of benzodiazepines in normal therapeutic doses (defined as up to 30 mg/day of diazepam or equivalent) for at least one year. Subjects who had never been prescribed a benzodiazepines or who had taken these drugs in the past for less than one year ($n=61$) were recruited from voluntary organizations and employment agencies. The group of subjects who had taken benzodiazepines continuously for at least one year and who had successfully withdrawn from their medication for at least six months ($n=34$) was obtained from both general practices and the outside agencies. No subject with a history of excessive alcohol use, epilepsy, brain injury, psychotic illness, cerebrovascular accident, or the use of monoamine oxidase inhibitors or antipsychotic drugs was included in the study.

We employed a wide range of tests to search for possible effects.

National Adult Reading Test (NART)

This reading test assesses premorbid intelligence in patients with dementia (18). In the present study, it was used to provide a measure of intellectual ability before the possible development of drug-related deterioration. The NART comprises a list of 50 words printed in order of increasing difficulty, all of which are 'irregular' with respect to the common rules of pronunciation. The subject was asked to read aloud down the list, and the number of pronunciation errors recorded.

Cancellation test

In this test of sustained attention, subjects were presented with a sheet of paper with rows of numbers containing forty 4s in 400 numbers (19). They were instructed to cancel out all the 4s, and the time taken was recorded.

Reaction time

Simple reaction time to identical visual stimuli, the number '1' presented on a computer screen was measured. After eight practice trials, the mean reaction time for 32 test trials was calculated.

Digit symbol substitution test

This subtest of the WAIS (20) is a coding task in which symbols are substituted for numbers. The score was the number of items correct in 90 seconds.

Symbol copying test

In this test of motor speed, the same symbols are used as in the digit symbol test, but the subject has only to copy and not code them (21). The score was the number of items correct in 90 seconds.

Block design

This sub-test of the WAIS (20) is a construction test which measures visual-spatial organization: subjects use red and white blocks to construct replicas of 9 red and white designs printed in smaller scale. One score is obtained for each subject, according to the speed and accuracy of completion of the designs.

Verbal recall memory

Forty-nine randomly ordered words were presented individually for two seconds, at two-second intervals (22). The word list comprised seven categories, with seven words in each. The categories were selected from those of Battig and Montague (23), and the words balanced across categories for frequency of use. Immediately the list had been presented, the subjects were instructed to write down as many of the words as possible in any order, in two minutes, and this procedure was repeated twice, using the same words in a different random order each time. The total number of words correctly recalled over the three trials was calculated. To provide a measure of delayed recall, the subjects were asked to write down as many words as they could remember 1½ hours later.

New learning

The ability to learn new material was assessed from the verbal recall test by subtracting the subject's score for trial 1 from the score for trial 3.

Visual spatial recognition memory

This is a computerized spatial recognition test (24). The subject memorizes a design, and then has to recognize that previously-seen design from a triad which includes two new designs. The interval between initial presentation of the stimulus and its re-appearance on the screen with two new designs is 1, 5, and 10 seconds. There are 36 trials altogether, with 12 at each of the three retention intervals; the total number correct and mean reaction time were scored.

Little men

This is a computerized measure of spatial orientation (24). A 'manikin' appears on the screen, holding a baton in one hand; he may be facing away from the subject, on his feet or on his head, and the baton may be in the right or left hand. Subjects are required to make a left/right discrimination for 32 trials; the total number of correct trials and mean response time were scored.

Visual perceptual analysis

This computerized measure of visual information-processing examines the subject's ability to perceive small differences in complex abstract designs (24). Three designs, two of which are identical, appear on the screen, and the subject has to indicate the different one. The test has 32 trials — 16 'hard' and 16 'easy'; total number correct and mean reaction time were scored.

Trail making

In this test of visual conceptual and visuomotor tracking (25), the subject was asked to draw lines to connect consecutively numbered circles on one work sheet (Trail Making A), and then to connect the same number of consecutively numbered and lettered circles on another work sheet by alternating between the two sequences (Trail Making B). Time taken in seconds to complete each part was recorded.

Bexley-Maudsley category sorting test

This computerized test has been adapted from the Wisconsin card sorting test (26,27,28). The subject is required to use abstract concepts to solve a problem, and to change concepts as the computer alters the criteria for solution of the problem. Four standard designs are presented, incorporating three dimensions—the orientation of the elements, the number of elements, and the type of elements. The subject has to assign serially presented test designs to one of the standard designs on the basis of orientation, number, or type, and is told after each trial whether or not the response was correct. The computer takes the subject through two cycles of these three concepts. The following scores were obtained: number of categories—total number of concepts achieved; total number of sorts to complete the test; total number of errors; and perseverations—number of errors which were repeated consecutively.

Controlled word association test

This measure of verbal fluency requires subjects to say as many words as they can think of which begin with the letter 'F' in 60 seconds, excluding proper nouns, numbers, and words with the same prefix. This procedure is then repeated with the letters 'A' and 'S' (29), and the sum of correct words in the three categories scored.

Cognitive Failures Questionnaire (CFQ)

This scale measures self-reported failures in perception, memory and motor function (30). The subject indicates the frequency with which he or she has made such mistakes in the past six months on a five point scale, ranging from 'never' to 'very often'. A total score is obtained by summing the score for each item.

State anxiety inventory

This scale provides a measure of the subject's level of anxiety at the time of testing. The subject rates 20 statements about how he or she feels at that particular moment on a four-point scale, ranging from 'not at all' to 'very much so' (31). A total score is obtained by summing the score for each item.

Benzodiazepine dosage

If anti-anxiety drug usage and neuropsychological deficits are associated, one would expect some dose, time, or (most likely) cumulative dose relationship. A global measure of benzodiazepine intake (BZG) was calculated for each subject by multiplying the length of time for which the subject had taken a particular benzodiazepine with its dose for each benzodiazepine taken, and then summing these scores. Length of time was measured in months and the dose was categorized as: less than the minimum therapeutic dose; maintenance dose; maximum therapeutic dose; and above the maximum therapeutic dose. Similarly, a global measure of antidepressant intake (ADG) was calculated.

Analysis of subjects still taking benzodiazepines and the matched control group

In selecting the sample, subjects with different levels of benzodiazepine intake were balanced for age, further education, and NART score, all of which affect test performance. Pearson product-moment correlation coefficients between each of these variables and BZG showed no significant relationship with benzodiazepine intake, confirming that the subjects had been successfully matched for age, number of years of further education, and NART score—the measure of premorbid IQ.

Correlations

Product-moment correlation coefficients between BZG and the test variables are shown in Table 2. Significant relationships were found for the cancellation test, digit symbol substitution, symbol copying, block design, new learning, little men, and visual perceptual analysis: subjects with a high previous benzodiazepine intake were impaired on these tests.

Multiple regression

Seven variables found to be significantly related to benzodiazepine intake were entered into a multiple regression analysis using stepwise extraction. Two factors were found

Table 2
Correlations between benzodiazepine intake and test variables

	Pearson's R	Significance
Cancellation test	0·23	$p<0·01$
Reaction time	0·10	NS
Digit symbol substitution	−0·27	$p<0·01$
Symbol copying	−0·19	$p<0·05$
Block design	−0·22	$p<0·01$
Verbal recall	−0·11	NS
Delayed recall	−0·12	NS
New learning	−0·23	$p<0·01$
Spatial recognition	−0·11	NS
Spatial recognition reaction time	0·05	NS
Little men	−0·22	$p<0·01$
Little men reaction time	0·11	NS
Visual perceptual analysis	−0·27	$p<0·01$
Visual perceptual analysis reaction time	0·09	NS
Trail making 'A'	0·14	NS
Trail making 'B'	0·09	NS
Bexley-Maudsley category sorting		
N of Categories	−0·03	NS
N of Sorts	0·05	NS
N of Errors	0·12	NS
Perseverations	0·17	NS
Word association	−0·03	NS
Cognitive failures questionnaire	0·14	NS

to be predictive of BZG. Factor 1 was characterized by visual perceptual analysis ($p<0.01$); there were indications from changes in significance levels that symbol copying, block design, and little men were closely related to this factor. Factor 2 was extracted with the cancellation test ($p<0.02$), and was related to digit symbol substitution and new learning.

State anxiety

Subjects could not be balanced for level of anxiety during testing, as those who had a high benzodiazepine intake were also the most anxious. State anxiety was significantly correlated with benzodiazepine intake at the 1% level, thus possibly obscuring the relationship between BZG and test performance. Correlations between

Table 3
Correlations between state anxiety and test variables

	Pearson's R	Significance
Cancellation test	−0.23	$p<0.05$
Reaction time	−0.02	NS
Digit symbol substitution	0.05	NS
Symbol copying	0.20	$p<0.05$
Block design	0.05	NS
Verbal recall	0.05	NS
Delayed recall	0.03	NS
New learning	−0.05	NS
Spatial recognition	−0.02	NS
Spatial recognition reaction time	−0.04	NS
Little men	0.05	NS
Little men reaction time	−0.12	NS
Visual perceptual analysis	0.02	NS
Visual perceptual analysis reaction time	−0.18	NS
Trail making 'A'	−0.11	NS
Trail making 'B'	−0.07	NS
Bexley-Maudsley category sorting		
N of Categories	0.18	NS
N of Sorts	−0.18	NS
N of Errors	−0.15	NS
Perseverations	−0.02	NS
Word association	−0.04	NS
Cognitive failures questionnaire	0.36	$p<0.001$

state anxiety and the tests themselves were found to be significant only for the cancellation test and the symbol copying test (Table 3). For both of these variables, the effect of state anxiety needs eliminating before interpreting any relationship with benzodiazepine intake. However, partial correlations controlling for state anxiety revealed a relationship between BZG and both the cancellation test ($r=0.5$; $p<0.01$) and the symbol copying test ($r=0.27$; $p<0.02$), after state anxiety had been removed. Not surprisingly, the most anxious subjects also had high scores on the cognitive failures questionnaire ($r=0.36$; $p<0.001$).

Antidepressants and short-term benzodiazepine effects

Of the product-moment correlation coefficients between antidepressant intake (ADG) and the 21 test variables, only one significant relationship was found—between ADG and digit symbol substitution ($r = 0.18$; $p < 0.05$). This is probably spurious, with no significant link between antidepressant intake and poor performance on the test battery. Similarly, our findings cannot be accounted for by the short-term effects of benzodiazepines. Only one variable, new learning ($p < 0.05$) was significantly correlated with the dose taken on the day of testing.

Analysis of subjects who had withdrawn from benzodiazepines

Patients who had withdrawn from medication proved elusive, and careful matching was feasible. They were compared with a group of patients still on medication to examine whether or not patients who stop taking benzodiazepines return to normal cognitive functioning. The subjects still on medication had significantly higher mean BZG score than those who had withdrawn. In order to balance the two groups for benzodiazepine intake, subjects with a high BZG score who were still taking these drugs were excluded. Subsequently, no significant differences in cognitive functioning were found between the groups. A further comparison between those who had withdrawn from medication and subjects who had never taken benzodiazepines also failed to show differences in performance.

Thus, the long-term use of benzodiazepines seems to be associated with two areas of cognitive impairment. The first is visual-spatial ability, as measured by visual perceptual analysis, symbol copying, block design, and little men. The second concerns attention or, more specifically, the ability to sustain attention on a repetitive task under time pressure, as shown by a deficit in performance on the cancellation test, the digit symbol substitution test and new learning. Global measures of intellectual functioning such as memory, verbal fluency, flexibility, and simple reaction time seemed unaffected. This pattern of impairment is consistent with deficits in posterior cortical cognitive function. The tests which showed impaired performance are those which are generally affected by parietal, posterior temporal, and occipital rather than frontal lesions (32). Why the drugs should be selective is unclear; research on the mode of action of benzodiazepines may be at too early a stage to explain the specificity of their effects on cognitive functioning.

Of course, the poor performance of long-term benzodiazepine users might be due to other factors which are common to these patients; in particular, the anxiety for which benzodiazepines are prescribed is associated with impaired performance on tests of cognitive ability. However, anxiety-related impairment was demonstrated for only two of the tests, and when the effects of anxiety had been accounted for, the deficit in performance remained. Moreover, if our findings could be explained by anxiety, we would expect poor performance on all of the tests, especially on high-demand tasks (33,34).

One cannot venture how long it is safe for a patient to continue to take benzodiazepines, or at what dose, before cognitive ability will begin to deteriorate. Nevertheless, our data suggest that taking a low dose for a short time has little effect, while a high intake is almost certainly harmful. As with alcohol, the effect is cumulative—the higher the intake, the greater the risk (35).

The comparison between subjects who had stopped taking benzodiazepines and those still on medication remains inconclusive. Those no longer taking these drugs had had a comparatively low intake of benzodiazepines and were, therefore, unlikely to have shown much impairment while on medication. The fact that our sample comprised only subjects with a low intake suggests that few of those with a high intake manage to withdraw.

Two of the three areas of cognitive functioning found to be impaired after short-term benzodiazepine administration (36) — the ability to perform simple repetitive tasks and the ability to learn new material — are also impaired after chronic medication. However, performance on a variety of memory tasks, the third area which is impaired after short-term administration, showed no obvious deficit for long-term users. In a review of the effects of benzodiazepines on memory, Curran (37) describes a close association between sedation and memory impairment. This would suggest that as patients become tolerant to the sedative effects of benzodiazepines, memory deficits would diminish, which may well explain why memory impairment found after short-term administration is not apparent in chronic users.

A major discrepancy between the short- and long-term effects of benzodiazepines is in visual-spatial ability. Lader (36) concluded that such a well-established higher mental function is not impaired by the short-term use of these drugs, yet poor visual-spatial ability was found to be the greatest problem among chronic users. The tests of visual-spatial performance in the present investigation appear, in general, to require more elaborate processing of information than those used in short-term studies. Benzodiazepines may interfere with complex perceptual analysis, rather than with simpler visual-perceptual skills; otherwise, it seems likely that deterioration of visual-spatial ability develops only after benzodiazepines have been taken for a long period of time.

The finding that patients taking high doses of benzodiazepines for long periods of time perform poorly on tasks involving visual-spatial ability and sustained attention, implies that these patients are not functioning well in everyday life. Furthermore, the lack of relationship between benzodiazepine intake and the cognitive failures questionnaire, a subjective measure of impairment, suggests that they are not aware of their reduced ability. This is in line with clinical evidence that patients who withdraw from their medication often report improved concentration and increased sensory appreciation, and that only after withdrawal do they realize that they had been functioning below par (16,38).

References

(1) Balter MB, Manheimer DI, Mellinger GD, Uhlenhuth EH. A cross-national comparison of antianxiety/sedative drug use. *Curr Med Res Opinion* 1984; **8** (Suppl 4): 5-20.
(2) Hindmarch I. Psychomotor function and psychoactive drugs. *Br J Clin Pharmacol* 1980; **10**: 189-209.
(3) Rickels K, Case G, Downing RW, Winokur A. Long-term diazepam therapy and clinical outcome. *JAMA* 1983; **250**: 767-71.
(4) Rickels K, Case WG, Downing RW, Winokur A. Indications and contraindications for chronic anxiolytic treatment: is there tolerance to the anxiolytic effect? In: Kemali D, Racagni G, eds. *Chronic treatments in neuropsychiatry*. New York: Raven Press, 1985, 193-204.
(5) Lucki I, Rickels K, Geller AM. Chronic use of benzodiazepines and psychomotor and cognitive test performance. *Psychopharmacology* 1986; **88**: 426-33.

(6) Aranko K, Mattila MJ, Bordignon D. Psychomotor effects of alprazolam and diazepam during acute and subacute treatment, and during the follow-up phase. *Acta Pharmacol Toxicol* 1985; **56**: 364–72.
(7) Aranko K, Mattila MJ, Nuutila A, Pellinen J. Benzodiazepines, but not antidepressants or neuroleptics, induce dose-dependent development of tolerance to lorazepam in psychiatric patients. *Acta Psych Scand* 1985; **72**: 436–46.
(8) Lader MH. Dependence on benzodiazepines. *J Clin Psych* 1983; **44**: 121–7.
(9) Fontaine R, Chouinard G, Annable L. Rebound anxiety in anxious patients after abrupt withdrawal of benzodiazepine treatment. *Am J Psych* 1984; **41**: 848–53.
(10) Robertson I. Does moderate drinking cause mental impairment. *Br Med J* 1984; **289**: 711–2.
(11) Bond AJ, James DC, Lader MH. Physiological and psychological measures in anxious patients. *Psychol Med* 1974; **4**: 364–73.
(12) Hendler N, Cimini C, Terence MA, Long D. A comparison of cognitive impairment due to benzodiazepines and to narcotics. *Am J Psych* 1980; **10**: 189–209.
(13) Johnson LC, Chernik DA. Sedative-hypnotics and human performance. *Psychopharmacology* 1982; **76**: 101–13.
(14) Bond AJ, James DC, Lader MH. Sedative effects on physiological and psychological measures in anxious patients. *Psychol Med* 1974; **4**: 374–80.
(15) Tansella M, Zimmermann-Tansella C, Lader M. The residual effects of N-desmethyldiazepam in patients. *Psychopharmacologia* 1974; **38**: 81–90.
(16) Petursson H, Gudjonsson GH, Lader MH. Psychometric performance during withdrawal from long-term benzodiazepine treatment. *Psychopharmacology* 1983; **81**: 345–9.
(17) Golombok S, Moodley P, Lader M. Cognitive impairment in long-term benzodiazepine users. *Psychol Med* 1987; in press.
(18) Nelson H. *The national adult reading test*. Windsor: NFER-Nelson, 1982.
(19) Kornetsky C, Vates TS, Kessler EK. A comparison of hypnotic and residual psychological effects of single doses of chlorpromazine and secobarbital in man. *J Pharmacol Exp Ther* 1959; **127**: 51–4.
(20) Wechsler D. *Wechsler adult intelligence scales: a manual*. New York: Psychological Corporation, 1955.
(21) Bond AJ, Lader MH. Residual effects of hypnotics. *Psychopharmacologia* 1972; **25**: 117–32.
(22) Curran HV, Shine P, Lader MH. Effects of repeated doses of fluvoxamine, mianserin and placebo on memory and measures of sedation. *Psychopharmacology* 1986; **89**: 360–3.
(23) Battig WF, Montague WE. Category norms for verbal items in 56 categories: a replication and extension of the Connecticut Category norms. *J Exp Psychol* 1969; **80**: 1–46.
(24) Acker W, Acker C. *Bexley-Maudsley automated psychological screening*. Windsor: NFER-Nelson, 1982.
(25) Reitan RM. Validity of the trail making test as an indicator of organic brain damage. *Percept Motor Skills* 1958; **8**: 271–6.
(26) Acker W, Acker C. Bexley-Maudsley category sorting test. Windsor: NFER-Nelson, 1982.
(27) Berg EA. A simple objective technique for measuring flexibility in thinking. *J Gen Psychol* 1948; **39**: 15–22.
(28) Grant DA, Berg EA. A behavioral analysis of degree of reinforcement and ease of shifting to new responses in a Weigl-type card sorting problem. *J Exp Psychol* 1948; **38**: 408–11.
(29) Benton AL. Differential behavioural effects in frontal lobe disease. *Neuropsychologia* 1968; **6**: 53–60.
(30) Broadbent DE, Cooper PF, Fitzgerald P, Parkes KR. The cognitive failures questionnaire (CFQ) and its correlates. *Br J Clin Psychol* 1982;. **21**: 1–16.
(31) Spielberger G, Gorsuch A, Lushene A. *Test manual for the state-trait anxiety inventory*. Palo Alto: Consulting Psychologists Press, 1970.
(32) Kolb B, Whishaw IQ. *Fundamentals of human neuropsychology*. San Francisco: WH Freeman & Co, 1980.

(33) Eysenck M. *A handbook of cognitive psychology.* London: Lawrence Erlbaum, 1984.
(34) Hockey R. Stress and the cognitive components of skilled performance. In: Hamilton V, Warburton D, eds. *Human stress and cognition: an information processing approach.* Chichester: John Wiley, 1979.
(35) Ron M. *The alcoholic brain: CT scan and psychological findings.* Cambridge: Cambridge University Press, Psychological Medicine Monograph Supplement 3. 1983.
(36) Lader MH. Benzodiazepines, psychological functioning and dementia. In: Trimble MR, ed. *Benzodiazepines divided.* Chichester: John Wiley, 1983: 309–325.
(37) Curran HV. Tranquillising memories: a review of the effects of benzodiazepines on human memory. *Biol Psychol* 1985; **23**: 179–213.
(38) Curran HV, Golombok S. *Bottling it up.* London: Faber & Faber, 1985.

Discussion

Asked if he had looked at the relationship between dosage and time, **Professor Lader** said that he had examined these two independently, and that the correlations were quite weak; what he had shown was the integral of the two.

Professor Rickels referred to the deficits shown in the chronic users and asked if the same was found later. **Professor Lader** said that if they took those who had withdrawn earlier, there were no deficits, but these were much lower users; the study had been cross-sectional, and chronic users were not re-tested. **Professor Rickels** had understood that in the 36 patients who had been off benzodiazepines for six months, the same results had not been found. **Professor Lader** agreed that there were no significant correlations, but reiterated that they had been the lighter users.

Dr File said that only 4% of the variance in Professor Lader's data was accounted for by the total benzodiazepine over time, but thought that the very heavy long-term users could be increasing the correlation coefficient. She also pointed out that alcohol intake could account for more than 4% of the variance.

Professor Lader said that 4% of between-subject variance was quite appreciable; the remaining 96% was individual variance. Although alcohol might be one of the factors influencing variance, they had excluded the heavy users, and the literature suggested that there was a threshold for alcohol use, though it was not very clearly defined. **Dr File** said that impairment of performance started at about a bottle of wine a week.

Professor Rickels asked whether an analysis of variance had been done on the three groups, and if the groups were significantly different from each other. **Professor Lader** replied that they had not done so because of the low numbers; the problem was that they could not balance these groups, since the light users did not show the same relationship.

Professor Rickels agreed with Dr File that it was, then, a chance finding, but **Professor Lader** replied that it was the heavy users who were bringing in the impairment. The criterion for inclusion was an intake of 30 mg/day, and those taking more than that equivalent at the time of testing were excluded. The interval between the last dose and the test had been at least 6 h. They had looked at the correlation between the dosage taken, the time after taking, and the test, and had found no relationship, so that there was no evidence that this was an effect of the last dose of benzodiazepines that had been taken. Plasma levels had not been measured.

General discussion

Professor Clare asked the Meeting to consider a number of points.

First, the suggestion that benzodiazepines should be removed from the list of prescribed drugs, and their sale across the counter permitted, their prevalence and use then to be controlled by the factors used currently to control alcohol—price, retail outlets, taxation, advertising, and general education.

Second, if the answer to the first point was 'no', should there be no change in usage, or should it be restricted to exceptional conditions such as epilepsy or chronic intractable anxiety?

Third, if there was not to be restriction to specific categories, what were the recommended indications for use?

Fourth, what guidelines could be drawn up with regard to their use?

Fifth, what alternative treatments could be suggested with regard to those conditions in which these drugs were either not indicated, or were not the treatment of choice?

Taking the first point, it had been suggested that alcohol and the benzodiazepines had remarkable similarities, and, given what was known about the benzodiazepines, should they be available in the community as alcohol was?

Dr Marks wished to emphasize that the regulations on the use of alcohol had been virtually dismantled, accounting in part for the current problems. Alcohol was controlled by fiscal measures, by limitation on the outlets, and by restrictions on the hours in which it was available, which had not been very rigorous until the First World War. Since the Second World War, the price in real terms had plummeted both for beer and spirits, and alcohol could be bought now at supermarkets at any time of the day.

Dr Christie said that in 1983/4, the State of Victoria, Australia, had passed legislation permitting the pharmacist to dispense up to ten capsules or tablets of either nitrazepam or tamezepam without prescription. A review of the situation was carried out about six months ago, and revealed no trouble arising from the practice, despite the dire predictions during months of debate prior to the legislation, and the fact that the pharmaceutical industry had opposed it. New South Wales had passed similar legislation, but it continued to be a controversial issue there.

Dr Williams thought it would be an act of extreme political naïveté, given the current climate of opinion about benzodiazepines, to recommend that they be freely available. The pharmaceutical industry did not want it, and it would be politically foolish if the medical profession were seen to be recommending it.

The benzodiazepines in current clinical practice, edited by Hugh Freeman and Yvonne Rue, 1987: Royal Society of Medicine Services International Congress and Symposium Series No. 114, published by Royal Society of Medicine Services Limited.

Professor Clare thought that although the instruments of control were available, the experience with alcohol indicated the difficulty of exercising that control.

Mr Taylor said that although the distribution of benzodiazepines was controlled by doctors, they obviously did not have absolute control over day-to-day use. As to price control, he did not think it unreasonable that some consumers should pay for their prescriptions.

Dr Marks felt that medical control was very haphazard, as evidenced by the black market in benzodiazepines, but the question was raised whether it would be less haphazard with pharmacists. He thought the patient should be the control—not the pharmacist or the doctor: the patient already determined what he or she did with the prescription—put it into a yew tree or actually bought the drugs. Because drugs were available across a counter, that did not necessarily mean that many people would actually go and buy them.

Dr Wells said that despite the fact that all doctors were not prescribing perfectly, it was still better for them to have that degree of medical control. The objective should be to improve prescribing rather than to deregulate the drugs; that would be politically unwise and not very sensible from other points of view.

Professor Clare said that there seemed to be general agreement that the present system of control should remain as it is.

So far as guidelines for the use of benzodiazepines were concerned, there were NIMH consensus recommendations concerning the prescribing of anxiolytics and hypnotics which were similar to the DSM III diagnostic categories.

Dr Christie pointed out that the Bethesda Conference had dealt only with sedative hypnotics, not their use as tranquillizers. However, **Professor Rickels** said that nevertheless, there were similarities.

Dr Imlah thought that one of the great problems in categorizing people by disorder was that people reacted differently. There was a very wide variation in response to benzodiazepines, and some people on long-term medication might continue to benefit from it.

Professor Lader pointed to the very wide range of opinions among psychiatrists on the indications for these drugs.

Professor Clare asked if guidelines could in fact be given with regard to the diagnostic categories, because individual patients and individual states differed. In teaching medical students, one started with conditions in which benzodiazepines were classically used, but were there also conditions in which they should never be used? Another view was that these were all-purpose drugs, to be used from time to time, depending on circumstances, timing, the characteristics of the patient, etc.

Dr Marks said he would not use it for panic disorder in the first instance; he would treat with psychological remedies primarily, and only give a benzodiazepine for a short period initially, to produce a state in which patients could cooperate with treatment.

Professor Rickels said that in the USA, where health care was not free, people did not want the expense of 12 weeks treatment by a therapist when they might be helped by only one or two weeks of benzodiazepines use. He thought that benzodiazepines were the cheapest and most effective remedy for many patients.

Dr Tyrer believed that insomnia was a symptom; if there was an underlying problem, one might use a benzodiazepine, but simply to treat insomnia symptomatically was inappropriate. Where events were related to the symptoms, benzodiazepines could be used, unless the experience of the event was psychologically important, i.e. if a patient was distressed because a close relative had died, it might be inappropriate to use a benzodiazepine and so perhaps promote denial of the psychological adjustment to the event. Anterograde amnesia in this situation was undesirable.

Dr File asked if he was saying that episodic anterograde amnesia would prevent the course of behaviour therapy or cognitive therapy: remembering that someone was dead was retrograde, and benzodiazepines would not affect that. She asked if there was any evidence that benzodiazepines would create problems in such a situation, but **Dr Tyrer** said there was none, because it was a very difficult thing to test. **Dr File** said that if the deficit was specific for episodic amnesia, and learning new skills was not impaired, she wondered whether the nature of the learning that the bereaved had to go through via some form of therapy was the kind of learning that benzodiazepines would impair.

Dr Tyrer said that for short-term use such as response to stressful events, which would be self-limiting, it was reasonable to think of using benzodiazepines. Where rapid onset of action was required, benzodiazepines should still be thought of before other drugs. On the other hand, if there were major symptoms in response to minor stresses or none at all, then those patients had the potential to go on to long-term use, and in that case, the treatment was more contentious. In conditions in which anxiety was a secondary symptom and there was no obvious cause, it took time to establish a diagnosis, but patients often wanted relief immediately. In that case promethazine, which could be bought over the counter might be useful, or else flupenthixol. If the condition persisted, then antidepressants could be considered; for several weeks' therapy one of these would be better than a benzodiazepine in alleviating the symptoms.

Dr File asked how one could be anxious to a psychologically unimportant stressful event; if one was anxious, was that not a definition of it being important? **Dr Tyrer** said it was psychologically important to face the stress: in psychological treatment, it becomes clear that denial of major life events and of the memory immediately afterwards produces a potentially explosive situation in the long-term, possibly resulting in more serious psychopathology. For that reason, he avoided benzodiazepines if it was important for the patient to face up to the event that had occurred. **Dr Beary** asked how he would advise a GP called to someone's death bed, to treat the grieving person. Would he deny them two or three nights' sleep? **Dr Tyrer** and **Dr Marks** both said that they would do so, in the first instance.

Professor Clare believed that general practice involved discussion between doctor and patient. Simply to deny the patient's request for medication was to return to the old style of general practice, in which the doctor always knew what was good for the patient.

Dr Higgs was concerned about rigid guidelines. To refuse to help somebody acutely distressed after their son had been killed in a motorcycle accident, where there had been no chance to prepare them for the death, seemed to him quite extraordinary. The skill of general practice lay in assessing whether or not a patient was going to be able to cope with the effect of bereavement in the acute event, or whether he would go completely to pieces, and then in determining exactly what prescription to give. Often, a very small prescription was adequate; more than 15 or 20 tablets seemed like long-term administration.

Professor Lader said that another dimension to consider was the simple one of severity. These drugs were indicated for the relief of severe symptomatic distress, where other measures were either inappropriate or ineffectual; cognitive therapy did not work with somebody who was severely shocked. Therefore, when one was using symptomatic remedies, severity was the most important dimension. **Professor Clare** thought that was a very helpful guideline as to certain circumstances in which benzodiazepines might be used.

Dr Wheatley pointed out that the half-life of a drug in the plasma might not bear any relationship to the duration of a particular pharmacological effect. The more that concentration/effect relationships were studied, the less closely did plasma concentrations correlate with simultaneous pharmacological effects. Also, there might be more than one action. Phenothiazines, for example, had an immediate sedative action and a delayed antipsychotic effect; the antidepressive drugs had an immediate anticholinergic effect and a delayed antidepressive action. Anxiolytic effects and hypnotic effects had been discussed as though they were the same, but he would be surprised if the effect on long-term mood in response to stress was necessarily the same mechanism, acting on the same part of the central nervous system as that which put the patient to sleep. He wondered which of the pharmacological and therapeutic actions of benzodiazepines were more closely related to plasma levels; from some of the evidence presented earlier, it did not seem that the therapeutic action of a drug was dictated primarily by a long or short half-life.

Professor Lader thought that in the drugs currently available, there were very few pharmacodynamic differences, but there were some pharmacokinetic correlations. By and large, a short-acting benzodiazepine, given in a single dose at night, was much less likely to have residual effects detectable the next morning than a long-acting compound. Apart from this, there was no real differences in their action.

Dr Wheatley suggested that where the patient was taking a single dose in the daytime, that would be an indication for as short-acting a compound as possible. However, **Professor Lader** said it was not so simple, because the pharmacokinetics were much more complicated than just elimination half-life. Diazepam in a single dose was a short-acting compound, with a very marked redistribution half-life; very little could be detected 3 or 4 h after a single dose. Because of that, it was an excellent hypnotic, leaving no hangover effect.

Dr Wheatley wondered whether diazepam taken every day for five days would produce a permanent steady state level in the blood. **Professor Lader** thought that a low amount on intermittent use would not do so, but it was very dosage-determined, as all effects were.

Dr Higgs raised the question of withdrawal from short-acting, as opposed to long-acting compounds; it appeared to be much more difficult in practice to get patients off the short-acting compounds. **Dr Tyrer** said that although one should be careful not to extrapolate from pharmacokinetic data, it was difficult not to do so, particularly when two of the major compounds — triazolam and lorazepam — had relatively short half-lives, and the compounds with fewer problems, such as nitrazepam, had long half-lives. Obviously, there were other aspects apart from the elimination half-life — speed of onset of action, for instance. **Dr File** agreed that pharmacokinetics were quite different in chronic use, as were the pharmacodynamics. In animals, she had looked at brain concentration and correlated it with behavioural effect; with an acute dose, it correlated completely. The more drug in the brain, the bigger the effect on all responses, but with chronic treatment, there was no correlation. She had also found drug effects persisting several hours after any drug was detectable in the brain, though it was not known what caused these long-term effects. Finally, withdrawal response could be demonstrated after one single administration of a drug. She emphasized that these were animal data.

Professor Lader did not think it easy to come to a conclusion about half-life and withdrawal, because there were many factors to consider. One benzodiazepine was more likely to produce dependence than another, but no studies had ever put people randomly on the different groups of benzodiazepines and followed them through. Secondly, there was no doubt that someone coming off a short-acting compound could be detected more easily — one only had to wait 48 h, instead of seven days. Then, there was 'weekend withdrawal', where someone took a drug for five days during the week, and would feel anxious on Sunday; this was due to withdrawal from a short-acting compound.

The problem was that almost all of the shorter-acting compounds were of high potency; he agreed that something was confusing the issue and that there were not enough data to be categorical. Oxazepam was a low-potency, medium-acting compound, which did seem to have a low incidence of attendant problems. But in Sweden, where oxazepam and diazepam were used in about equal amounts, break-ins to chemists shops showed that three times as much diazepam was stolen as oxazepam, suggesting there were differences not related to usage.

Dr Imlah agreed that people could become dependent on almost all drugs, but in practice, it was easiest to withdraw them by transferring to oxazepam, and then withdrawing it. **Professor Lader** pointed out that another low-potency compound was chlordiazepoxide, with which there were fewer problems than with diazepam. There was therefore an indication that potency was equally or perhaps more important than half-life. By 'potency' he meant clinical dosage. However, **Dr File** said it was really a question of whether the drug had a low affinity for the receptor. There were data to suggest that oxazepam could be a partial agonist, and that might be a very important clue to finding a compound that was different in its profile. Potency was a loose term, and it was necessary to know whether it was affinity or partial agonist action that influenced the level of efficacy. **Professor Lader** said that these were low-ceiling efficacy compounds. The evidence was that oxazepam was not a very 'powerful' anxiolytic clinically; a high dose had low clinical potency. **Dr Tyrer** asked if it would be wrong to say that a drug which was effective in low doses had a greater affinity for the receptors. **Dr File** said it would not, but what was interesting was not its affinity, but whether it was a partial agonist.

Professor Turner said that if it was true that oxazepam had less efficacy, produced less changes in receptor population than other benzodiazepines, and therefore was less likely to produce withdrawal, then a positive guideline to general practitioners might be to switch patients from their present medication to oxazepam, as an intermediate step during withdrawal.

Professor Rickels said that some centres in the United States which had big problems with patients on long-term tranquillizers had transferred patients to oxazepam, and then tried to withdraw them. However, they had encountered withdrawal problems — much more so than with compounds with a long half-life. **Dr Tyrer** said that his group was undertaking a similar project, and the first part was to change over to a different benzodiazepine, given in equally efficacious doses; they were finding that it was actually very difficult to effect the change from one benzodiazepine to another.

Professor Clare thought it was also important to discuss the duration of treatment. Where at one time four weeks did not seem to predict long-term use, now he sensed the feeling was that one or two weeks was as safe as one could go, and then there should be a review. **Dr Higgs** felt that a month's prescription in general practice should be considered a long one; they should deal mainly with periods of between five days and a fortnight. However, **Professor Clare** thought it likely that some general practitioners regularly gave monthly prescriptions. **Dr Wells** said that it was important in starting a patient on benzodiazepines that they were not given a month's prescription *ab initio*. Some doctors did so, but it was important to emphasize that this was not appropriate prescribing. **Dr Wheatley** emphasized they were only talking about guidelines, and there would always be individual cases where the guidelines would not be followed.

Professor Rickels thought it was even more important that contact with the patient should be maintained; if a patient needed longer-term treatment, he should be monitored carefully, and reassessed before any further decisions were made.

Dr Imlah believed that any substance given continuously over four weeks had a risk of causing withdrawal symptoms; whether drugs were given for four weeks or four years, the important point was to withdraw patients slowly from them.

Professor Clare turned to the question of those people who were using benzodiazepines for the first time. **Dr Higgs** said that the reason most people took short-term diazepam was to enable them to come to terms with a temporary crisis; it was to enable them to regain control of their situation. **Dr Williams** said that if new prescribing of benzodiazepines had decreased, then clearly it was a pool into which there was not going to be much recruitment. However, **Professor Lader** said that increased selectivity could mean that doctors were not putting people on to benzodiazepines who would not have gone into that pool in any case.

Mr Taylor pointed out that it was the charged prescriptions that had decreased in number, which identified younger, employed people. Since the middle 1970s, the number of first prescriptions had remained constant in the UK, compared with the number of repeats. Two things seemed to be happening — the number of people first taking benzodiazepines was probably dropping, and because of this, the pool of long-term users was being whittled away. It would be useful, though, to know what problems people thought they were using the drugs for, and to have detailed knowledge of the pattern of consumption in the population. With that information, one could try to get some measure of outcome, relative to other possible interventions, and to identify the most cost-effective intervention. Society had only limited resources, but it was not possible up to now to say whether psychological therapy was better than giving benzodiazepines for short periods. There were not enough data to make clear decisions, and no-one seemed to be investing the money necessary to improve this process.

Professor Turner referred to the Exeter study which had finished at the end of 1986 (*Br J Pharm Pract* 1986; **8**: 359–63); its results suggested that in the elderly, at least twice the number of patients were on hypnotics who needed to be. **Professor Rickels** said that anyone, elderly or not, on regular hypnotics should be carefully monitored. **Dr Higgs** said that for many elderly and sleepless patients, the night was a dreadful thing, yet the Exeter results suggested that it was possible to remind people that they could sleep naturally.

Professor Clare asked what was wrong about an elderly person being maintained on a hypnotic drug. **Dr Beary** mentioned reports of people falling and breaking their hips as a result of being over-sedated. **Professor Lader** said that people on a nightly hypnotic could become progressively more intoxicated; there was a gross over-representation of fractured femurs amongst old women with osteoporosis who were taking benzodiazepines, whereas if such people were properly monitored, and the dose reduced as they became more sensitive, these problems could be lessened.

Professor Turner replied that this was very controversial: a recent paper had suggested that the early work in Nottingham could not be repeated. (Rashiq S, Logan RFA. *Br Med J* 1986; **292**: 861–3.)

Professor Clare pointed out the difficulties that general practitioners would experience in monitoring very large numbers of elderly patients who were taking nightly hypnotics.

Dr Higgs said he normally ensured that he never prescribed beyond three months without seeing elderly patients, but he preferred to see them every month. Many GPs were not giving enough thought to getting people off their drugs, and the paradoxical situation arose where patients wanted to come off the drug; the doctor was giving it to them; they were angry about that, and the person they needed help from most in order to get off the drug was their doctor. Therapeutic groups were an advantage in the withdrawal situation, because patients supported each other through the period of withdrawal. **Dr Williams** had found that when long-term users were asked 'what is your doctor's view about long-term use', the most common response was 'I don't know'. **Professor Clare** suggested that every patient using these drugs should know clearly their doctor's view of both short- and long-term use.

Dr Wells said that when drugs were given in the first place, it should be pointed out that they were a means to an end, not an end in themselves. **Dr Marks** added that it was also necessary to educate the specialists, otherwise the situation could arise where the GP referred a patient to a specialist, and the specialist recommended continuing the drug. **Dr Wheatley** pointed out that although patients may want to stop the drugs, they may also want some substitute for the effects that the drug was having. If they experienced adverse effects on withdrawal, it was likely that they would simply start taking the drugs again, and doctors could often offer no alternative.

Dr File returned to the question of whether tolerance to a drug's effects and the withdrawal responses were linked. The evidence suggested that if tolerance to a drug's effects could be shown, then withdrawal responses could also be shown; if one could not show tolerance, then one could not get withdrawal. If a patient had withdrawal responses, it therefore suggested that they had become tolerant to that drug's effects, in which case they would not need a substitute for the drug, because the drug had ceased to have an effect. **Dr Wheatley** referred specifically to the use of hypnotics in the elderly: old people slept more irregularly than the young, and this was adverse for them psychologically. If they were withdrawn from their drug, their insomnia returned; he did not know what to do about that. **Dr File** said that patients may well become tolerant to the effects of benzodiazepines, and that the drugs were no longer changing their sleep pattern. **Dr Wheatley** pointed out that patients were still sleeping well on continued benzodiazepines, but **Dr Higgs** wondered if this could be a placebo effect. **Professor Turner** said that he would not argue about tolerance in the case of centrally acting benzodiazepine drugs, but he did not think that a statement should be made that if withdrawal occurs to a drug, this meant that tolerance to the drug had developed.

Dr Marks thought it was important from the clinical point of view that doctors got elderly people off benzodiazepines, helped them over their withdrawal symptoms, and returned to a situation where they were not using a benzodiazepine, and yet did not perceive a shortened sleep as distressing. **Dr Beary** suggested that before a hypnotic was prescribed to elderly people, they should be informed that their physiology changed as they grew older, and that their total sleep did not decline, but was broken throughout the day. An afternoon nap might well be the answer to their problem, rather than a drug. **Professor Clare** pointed out that many GPs were currently doing precisely that. **Dr Wheatley** also agreed that the physiological reduction in sleep requirement in the elderly might be compensated by daytime napping, but it remained a fact that the long period of darkness for an old person alone could be very distressing. The doctor's job was to relieve distress, and if that entailed prescribing a benzodiazepine or other hypnotic, then he considered it to be justified. As in every other clinical situation, however, the possible harm the drug might do should be balanced against the harm of an illness left untreated. It was a matter of clinical judgment.

Professor Clare asked the Meeting to consider alternative treatments.

Dr Higgs said that every GP should, as part of his armamentarium, have access to a community psychiatric nurse, a psychologist, a counsellor, or a therapeutic group. So far as drug alternatives were concerned, a great many other drugs did not seem as safe as the benzodiazepines. **Dr Marks** again mentioned his experience of a successful scheme run by community psychiatric nurses in treating benzodiazepine addiction and phobic anxiety. Problems might arise in cases of withdrawal through a lack of straightforward behavioural techniques in departments of psychiatry, or in general practice where there was insufficient personnel. Community psychiatric nurses were more efficient, he had found, than psychologists, because the latter tended to treat on a one-to-one basis, and quickly filled up their case load; patients then had to wait for months before treatment.

Dr Higgs agreed that if someone was motivated, one could not afford to wait until later. **Dr Tyrer** said he had found a lot of goodwill and keenness amongst CPNs, but that appropriate skills were in short supply for problems such as this.

Professor Clare asked whether the present state of attachment of psychiatrists to primary care had any implications for the prescribing of benzodiazepines.

General discussion

Dr Beary said he had worked in a group practice for three years, and that one of his aims had been to confront this issue. The first thing was to have everybody who was on a repeat prescription seen every month, and that in itself reduced the number by approximately 40%. Having a list of the patients drawn up by the practice nurse seemed in itself to be a very effective measure, and just that pressure on the GP seemed to have dramatically reduced the repeat prescriptions.

Dr Higgs said that the impact on the medical team of having someone available to be involved in discussions on difficult patients or other problems could be considerable.

Chairman's summing up

ANTHONY CLARE

Department of Psychological Medicine,
St Bartholomew's Hospital Medical College, London EC1A 7BE, UK

One of the first things that emerges from this Symposium is that the benzodiazepines are regarded as a significant group of drugs, that needs to be regarded with considerable seriousness. Perhaps this is one of the consequences of the past ten years, during which time they were used in a rather cavalier way, not monitored, not audited, not particularly well studied. There have been several questions, however, which we have not been able to answer with any degree of agreement, because there is a great deal of information which is not yet available.

But there would appear to be agreement that it is reasonable to prescribe these drugs in an acutely stressful situation to enable the patient to regain control and then to cope, insofar as is possible, without them. Therefore, the severity and distress of the symptom and the disturbance caused by it are major factors determining prescribing. There seems to be agreement too that the shorter their use the better, but our group were not very willing to commit themselves on how long is a safe period of use, that is to say what is the largest dose and for how long can a benzodiazepine be prescribed without running severe risks. For a first prescription, it was generally felt that after 1-2 weeks there should be a review, and perhaps a period without drugs to assess the situation, before proceeding further.

This group came to the conclusion that the current pool of chronic users is not necessarily an expanding one, that it will reduce in size, and that perhaps it could be further reduced by more intense intervention such as the auditing of repeat prescriptions by general practitioners and greater concern on the part of doctors generally with regard to the use of these drugs.

There were no specific guidelines either about the use of short-acting versus long-acting drugs, though there was interest in the precise distinction between short and long, between hypnotic and tranquillizer, between potency and efficacy. There is always considerable agreement in such discussions about alternative treatments in general practice: i.e. that there should be better use of the consultation, a wider involvement of para-professionals or alternative professionals in primary care, such as health visitors, community psychiatric nurses, psychologists, and social workers. This group added its voice to that plea. However, the persistent reply from primary care is still the pressure on time, the fact that these drugs are cheap, that they are easy to prescribe, and that the great majority of the patients who use them

---

The benzodiazepines in current clinical practice, edited by Hugh Freeman and Yvonne Rue, 1987: Royal Society of Medicine Services International Congress and Symposium Series No. 114, published by Royal Society of Medicine Services Limited.

use them properly. Interestingly, this last point constitutes the great defence by the alcohol industry of alcohol: the vast majority of people drink sensibly. And the vast majority of benzodiazepine users take them sensibly.

We might ask why GPs are so stupid as to go on prescribing them. But then why are we so stupid as to go on drinking? The answer is that most of us know we get away with it. Most GPs get away with it; most patients get away with it, and those few who don't, end up as repeat prescribees. Most GPs do not even see them: the patients just come into the surgery, collect their prescription, and go away. They thereby relieve the GP of feeling any residual guilt about what he or she has done. That is something the group clearly wanted to change, but it was aware of the pressures on primary care doctors and indeed on patients which make them reach for these drugs. They are available, they are cheap, and—certainly in their initial phases—effective, whereas all the other alternatives take rather more time and mobilization of scarce resources.

It seems that the main conclusion at this stage is that there are still worrying reasons why we should regard the benzodiazepines as a good deal more potentially toxic and certainly more potentially hazardous than had been the case in the 1960s when they were introduced, and in the early 1970s when they were widely used. But the group was reluctant to provide hard-and-fast guidelines, for the very good reason that one cardinal truth about these drugs is that there are a variety of quite different circumstances in which one can make a very good case for using them, at least in the short term.

This meeting has provided an opportunity to review what little is known that is useful for clinicians in the field, who are battling with disease, stress, and disorder, and for outlining some of the areas of further fruitful research that might be undertaken. I personally will continue to think of ways in which at least one or two of these fairly modest questions about use and abuse, about persistence and duration, might be further clarified.